# *Dear Michael*

## Sexuality Education for <u>Boys Ages 11-17</u>

Cynthia G. Akagi

GYLANTIC PUBLISHING COMPANY
Littleton, Colorado

D1384236

Although the author has done research to ensure the accuracy and completeness of the information and drawings contained in this book, the author and publisher assume no responsibility for errors, inaccuracies, omissions, or any other inconsistency herein. Data contained herein are the most complete and accurate available as this book goes to press. Please bear in mind that meanings can vary due to personal interpretation.

To order additional copies:

GYLANTIC PUBLISHING COMPANY
P.O. Box 2792
Littleton, Colorado 80161-2792
1-800-828-0113
Add $2.00 to each order of less than four books for shipping and handling

Printed in the United States by Gilliland Printing, Inc.
The text is printed with soy ink.

Copyright © 1996 by Cynthia G. Akagi

Trademarks
Depo-Provera® is the trademark of The Upjohn Co., Kalamzoo, MI
Norplant System® is the trademark of Wyeth-Ayerst, Philadelphia, PA

Library of Congress Cataloging-in-Publication-Data

Akagi, Cynthia G., 1959-
    Dear Michael : sexuality education for boys ages 11-17 / Cynthia G. Akagi.
        p.   cm.
    Includes bibliographical references and index.
    Summary: A mother's letters to her son about puberty, girls, dating, sexual diseases, birth control, teen pregnancy, sexual abuse, and marriage.
        ISBN 1-880197-16-2 (alk. paper)
        1. Sex instruction for boys. 2. Sex instruction for teenagers.
[1. Sex instruction for boys.  2. Sex instruction for youth.]
I. Title.
HQ41.A38  1996
613.9'53—dc20                                    96-21271
                                                     CIP
                                                      AC

To CJ and Cory

# Acknowledgements

To the following people I extend many thank yous. This book would not have been possible without their assistance and support: my husband and children; illustrators Angie Di Cicco and Wanda Heberling; Juanita L. Smith, Director, Shawnee County Teen Pregnancy Prevention Program, Topeka, KS.; Dr. Betsy M. Bergen, sexuality professor, Kansas State University, Manhattan, KS; Jane Shirley, R.N., B.S.N. Jefferson County Health Department, Oskaloosa, KS; Todd Britt, family life educator, Winfield, KS; Georgia Balint, sexuality educator and her students, Topeka West High School, Topeka, KS; the mother/son critique teams which space doesn't allow me to list individually; my Wednesday night writing colleagues; the many friends who shared their teen memories with me; the Creator for the gift of writing.

# Table of Contents

# Foreword

Sometimes parents want to talk to their children about sexual issues but they don't know how or where to begin. Parents may feel uncomfortable because they were not taught by their parents. Today's parents may feel unsure and believe they are poorly equipped to communicate sexuality information to their children.

Now it is more important than ever that our children receive accurate and timely information concerning matters of human sexuality. The sexual revolution of the previous generation has given way to a far more dangerous place. In the era of AIDS, herpes, and other sexually transmitted diseases, casual and careless sex can ruin a life or even be fatal. Furthermore, the incidences of sexually transmitted diseases among adolescents and the number of teenage pregnancies are at an all time high. Sexuality education at an early age may be one way to combat these undesirable trends.

Cynthia Akagi has produced a unique tool in *Dear Michael* to help us communicate with our children. It is a series of letters, lovingly written from a mother to her son. The letters cover a wide variety of topics, including bodily changes during puberty, the feelings of love vs. lust, dating, romance, birth control, sexually transmitted diseases, relationships, and marriage.

Any letter can stand alone as a separate discussion, or it can be read in sequence with the entire series. The presentation is straightforward, easy to understand, and honest but never judgmental or preachy. Parents and their sons may read the letters together or as many boys would prefer, they can read the letters in the privacy of their own space. Questions are encouraged and space is provided at the end of each letter for boys to write down their questions or comments.

The information provided in *Dear Michael* is presented within a structure of the underlying major messages—we are all sexual beings, sexual feelings are a normal part of life, our bodies and feelings deserve to be treated with dignity and respect. Ms. Akagi also consistently emphasizes that sex is a serious matter and should be approached with responsibility and preferably within a framework of a lifelong commitment to another human being.

If you are a parent who wants your teenager to develop healthy and responsible attitudes about sexuality and especially if you are too embarrassed or uneasy about communicating with your son about sexuality, this book is for you. Read it and pass it on.

*Dear Michael* follows the publication of an equally excellent and candid book for girls entitled *Dear Larissa*, written as a series of letters from a mother to her daughter. I hope that many families read and share both volumes. These letters are a unique and valuable approach to sexuality education whether you are a father, daughter, mother, or son.

      Greggory J. Van Sickle, MD
      Topeka, Kansas

# Author's Note

When researching this book, the most often repeated comments I heard from sons regarding their parents were: "Although I'd never tell them this, my parents should have talked to me about sex earlier than they did. Even if I rolled my eyes and never said anything, I was hearing what they had to say. Parents don't realize what it's like to be a guy, and about aggressive girls who won't take no for an answer, and how early all this sexual stuff starts."

On the flip side, parents said: "It's hard accepting the fact that our boy is becoming a man. It seems like yesterday that he hated girls. Today he likes the sex he sees in advertising and on TV. We want him to know that sex is emotional and not just physical. We want him to know how to handle girls chasing him. We want him to know the seriousness of teen pregnancy, AIDS, and other sexually transmitted diseases."

For many of us talking to our sons is difficult. The birth control and teen pregnancy information in this book has been explained in a context suitable for pre-teens. Some parents may think: "I can't give my eleven year-old birth control information and talk to him about intercourse and pregnancy." If we want to impress upon our sons the seriousness of teen pregnancy, the message should begin at the pre-teen level. If we wait until our sons are sixteen to talk to them, they will have already formed their beliefs about having sex.

Some aspects of dating have changed since I was a teen and some things are still the same. So readers would know what other teens today think about dating, sex and love, I interviewed teens and included their comments.

I hope this book will be a good beginning for both of you. I hope you'll share it with other sons and parents.

---

This book is written from a heterosexual perspective. However, researchers estimate that about one in ten males is homosexual. If, during high school, your son *is not* interested in girls and dating *it does not mean he is homosexual.*

If you suspect your son is gay, or if he drops hints that he is gay, there are two things you can do for both of you:

(1) Continue to love and support your son, he is the same person you gave birth to. (2) If you don't know much about homosexuality, educate yourself. Consult the reading list in the back of this book and contact your library, county health department, family planning clinic, or family doctor for additional books and videos.

The national organization, Parents, Families, and Friends of Lesbians and Gays (PFLAG) provides support to parents of homosexual sons and daughters. To see if there is a local chapter in your area, you may call or write the national PFLAG office at 1012 14th Street, N.W., Suite 700, Washington, DC, 20005, (202) 638-4200.

# LETTER 1

# DEAR MicHAEl

Dear Michael,

You may be thinking. . . "Mom is giving me a book about sex?"

I'm giving you this book because you need information about sex and love, body changes, and dating and relationships.

Your teen years can be some of the best times of your life, but they can also be trying times. You'll be shaping who you are as a person. You'll be learning about relationships, dating, sex, and love. Because I was once a girl, I can answer questions you may have about girls.

Your dad and I could never give you all the sexuality information you need in one sitting, nor could you remember it all. One way to give you information is to write it down. You can read these letters in private and have time to think about the information.

Maturing into adulthood is about taking responsibility for your body and forming a set of personal values about your sexuality.

1

You may like dating and girls. You may go through a period where you hate girls. You may be having so much fun in school that you don't "seriously" fall in love until your twenties. Look at the guys in your class: some guys like girls, other guys don't care about dating yet.

The majority of people in your school are heterosexual and girls and guys want to date each other. But some males and females are homosexuals. They are attracted to people of their own sex. We'll talk about heterosexuality and homosexuality in Letter 3.

In terms of body changes and teen sex and love, you will learn more in your teens than at any other time in your life. That's why it's important for you to have the facts about growing up.

With correct information, you can make responsible decisions about sex and dating. Without correct information you can make a girl pregnant and become a teen father or catch sexually transmitted diseases (STDs) including AIDS, for which there is no cure. Having the facts will enable you to enjoy your teen years and have control over your body.

Michael, please know that you can come to me or your dad with any question or problem—even if it's embarrassing to you. Males who don't have contact with their dads can go to uncles, grandfathers, coaches, or other adult males they respect.

These letters should help us both feel more comfortable talking with each other and the book will be good reference information for you throughout high school.

Some of the information in these letters you won't need until you're older. You can refer back to that information when you need it. But because of the peer pressure teens face today, I want to give you all the facts now.

Here's to you and your teen years—school, friends, life!

I love you,
Mom

_____

_____

_____

_____

_____

_____

_____

_____

_____

# LETTER 2

# A History of Sex
# Since Grandpa Was a Teen

Dear Michael,

Before I talk about sex, love and dating, it's important that I share some of the history of sex education in your family and in America. It will help you understand why it's important that you and I talk about sexuality issues.

In your grandpa's day, sex was not discussed in most American homes. Before the 1980s, it also was not taught in most schools, except for the "menstruation film" for girls and maybe a short anatomy lesson in gym for the guys.

Our society was uncomfortable talking about sex. Teens were regarded as children, not as developing, sexual persons. Though teens had normal sexual feelings, they were often made to believe those feelings were wrong or dirty. Few teens were told that maturing into their adult bodies was a normal, healthy growth process.

In the fifties and early sixties many girls and guys did not have intercourse until they married. Boys were afraid of making a girl pregnant and for good reason. Reliable birth control was generally not available to unmarried males or females and abortions were illegal and dangerous. If a guy and girl did have sex and the girl became pregnant, they either married, or the girl was sent away to a relative where she had the baby and gave it up for adoption.

In 1960 a group of doctors created the oral contraceptive popularly known as "the pill." The pill was the first birth control that was 97% reliable for females. With the pill couples could postpone pregnancy until they were ready to be parents. Unfortunately, the sixties also introduced the idea of casual sex to society—if you like someone, have sex with them.

Parents knew that because of sexual diseases, teen pregnancy, and the emotional feelings of intimacy, casual sex was dangerous. But most parents were uncomfortable talking to their teens about sex. The only thing Grandpa told your dad was, "Don't stick your penis in anybody you wouldn't marry." The only information I received from Grandma was a warning to stay a virgin until I married.

If only Grandma and Grandpa had felt comfortable enough to sit down and explain that "yes, some people have sex before marriage, but there are risks." There are big risks like pregnancy, AIDS and other sexually transmitted diseases—as young people of the sixties and seventies found out. There are also emotional and self-respect issues—like a person using another person for sex and then dumping the person—and that happens a lot.

With little sexuality information being taught in the home or at school, most teens learned about sex by experimenting.

Experimenting is the wrong way to learn. Guys didn't understand that without birth control protection—even having sex one time—a girl could become pregnant. Many girls became pregnant. Neither sex was comfortable talking to each other about birth control.

Michael, your world is different today. Thankfully, society is realizing that teens are maturing young adults. You need to know about body changes, love, and sex so you can make responsible choices and avoid pregnancy, STDs, AIDS, and emotional pain.

Today, STDs affect one out of every three teens, in both country and city schools.

Your world can be terrifying. One wrong choice and you could become a teen father or contract AIDS or other STDs. That's why it's vital that you have the sexuality information you need to make responsible decisions for yourself when you begin dating.

Happily, I can give you this book and you can come to me or your dad with any type of question and I'll answer it for you.

Hugs,

Mom

_____

_____

_____

_____

_____

_____

_____

_____

_____

# LETTER 3

# YOUR CHANGING BODY AND CHANGING FEELINGS

Dear Michael,

It is quite miraculous the way our bodies change from child bodies to adult bodies. Physically, you'll grow body hair, your chest, scrotum and penis will develop, your voice will change, you'll begin shaving, and you'll have wet dreams (nocturnal emissions) and spontaneous erections.

Females also change. Girls develop breasts, their hips widen, they grow body hair, and begin menstruating (having periods). These physical changes are called "puberty." Puberty normally takes place between ten and sixteen years of age, but each person begins puberty according to his or her body's own time table.

Hormones (chemical messengers from your brain) begin the change toward adulthood. They signal your body to start equipping you with the physical capability to one day father children. The word puberty means "capable of reproduction."

When your body begins changing, you may feel somewhat uncomfortable or self-conscious. Changes are happening to

9

your body and you have no control over them. Body hair appears. You have your first wet dream. Help!

Michael, you're not alone. Every male feels a little weird and self-conscious when his body begins developing. Your dad told me he was in the sixth grade when he discovered he was growing pubic hair. At first he didn't even tell his best friend. What's tough is if, in comparison to your friends, you either mature early or late and you don't feel you fit in. If you are ever sitting in class worrying about yourself, look around the room. Everyone goes through the same body changes you are going through.

Maturing into your sexual adult body is a natural, healthy process. There is nothing dirty or bad about your body changing. During puberty your body's sexual hormones awaken so that as an adult you can enjoy and nurture a mature relationship through physical touch and someday have children.

To understand your new body, you need to look at yourself. You may want to study yourself in a mirror. Being familiar with your body will enable you to take care of your body, and there is nothing embarrassing about taking care of yourself.

After you read this letter, if you want to talk about a particular body change or you have questions about body growth, ask me. If I don't know the answers to your questions, I'll help you find the answers.

Preteen males are mostly concerned with body changes, wet dreams, and masturbation. Later on, guys are concerned about sexual feelings and how to understand girls. We'll discuss sexual feelings and girls in detail, but first things first.

Whatever feelings you first have—excited, anxious, self-conscious—any of those feelings are okay. Everyone who has experienced puberty has had all or some of those feelings. How do you feel right now? How do your friends feel about their changing bodies?

While your body is maturing, Michael, your emotions and thought processes are also maturing. You want to be part of the crowd, yet you want to be your own person. You want responsibility, but you don't want responsibility. You feel one way about a person or issue today, and tomorrow you totally change your mind. You want to do things by yourself and on your own, but you also want someone around if life becomes difficult.

This emotional maturing is called "adolescence," your mental maturing into adulthood. Adolescence lasts for several years, normally from age eleven through your early twenties. Adolescence is a critical growth process. It's the process by which you shape your adult personality, your values and goals, and how you'll interact with others as an adult.

Unfortunately, during adolescence, hormones working on your body development also affect your mental state. That's why teens can be moody—slight mood changes as well as serious mood swings. It's important to understand that many mood changes are due to hormones. It's equally important to work through those moods and feelings. You can write thoughts out in a journal, talk with a friend, and I'm here if you want to talk to me.

If you feel extremely blah, tired, sad, or brooding, you should talk with a school counselor, therapist, or doctor. Physical or emotional problems can cause depression. Your mental health is as important as your physical health. One can affect the other.

In addition to physical and emotional growth, you will also experience new sexual feelings.

Sexual adolescence can be broken down into three stages.

In *stage one* (grade school) you begin discovering the sexual world around you. You may like dirty jokes and become curious about the sex and love you see on television and in the movies. In grade school I remember leafing through clothing catalogs looking at the men's and women's underwear sections. Your uncle said that in the seventh grade he became infatuated with women's breasts.

At some time during the first and second stages of sexual adolescence children and preteens may play "doctor" with the same sex (two girls together, two boys together). These games are a normal expression of sexual curiosity. Playing them as a child or preteen does not mean you are a homosexual or an over-sexed person.

In the *second stage* of sexual awakening (junior high/middle school) you may become even more curious about sex, relationships, and dating. Some males want to date while others are still shy or unsure about dating. How do you feel?

About this time, girls are also experiencing a sexual awakening. Some girls want to date, literally chasing guys around. Other girls are in love with their favorite movie star or singer. Girls generally like romance and are as curious about the male body as you are about the female body.

The *final stage* of adolescent sexual awareness comes in high school. Your body is almost fully developed. Your sexual feelings are more intense. You may think about sex often, then wonder if you think about it too much. Nothing is wrong.

The following are sexuality questions we each try to answer at different times during our lives.

- Am I awkward looking? Do I look okay? Am I masculine?

- Do I think about sex a lot? Do I not care about sex much right now? Both feelings are normal.

- What are my sexual beliefs and values? What do I think about people making out? What do I think about intercourse?

- What do I think about my sexual identity? Am I tough, caring, or a mixture of both?

- Am I heterosexual (attracted to females) or homosexual (attracted to my own male sex)?

The majority of girls and guys in your school will be heterosexual—attracted to the other sex. But some people are homosexual. They are attracted to people of their own sex.

Homosexual men are called gays. Homosexual women are called lesbians, though the word "gay" is sometimes used to describe both homosexual men and women. You can't tell if someone is gay merely by their looks or how they act. A macho-male sports hero or a beautiful female model could be homosexual. Some researchers believe that homosexuality is a genetic manifestation (we are born heterosexual or homosexual). Other researchers believe that social environment and family influence sexual orientation. Homosexual men that I've talked to said that from early in their childhood they knew they were not heterosexual. The religious community is also divided on this issue of homosexuality. Some religions accept homosexuality. Other religions reject homosexuality.

Except for their sexual orientation, homosexuals are people like you and me. Gays have families, friends, talents, dreams, goals, successes, and disappointments. They work in sports, government, industry, religion, the arts, teaching, and the medical community. However, some people don't accept gays and lesbians as equal human beings.

School is especially tough on teens who think they may be homosexual. They wonder if they should act "straight" (heterosexual) because everyone else is into girl-guy dating. They often feel alone, isolated, and confused. Many homosexual teens don't feel safe talking to their friends or their parents for fear of being shunned, teased, and rejected.

But homosexual teens shouldn't be shunned. If you suspect someone in your circle of friends may be homosexual you could be a friend he or she can talk with. If you are uncomfortable being around homosexual people, you don't have to be best friends with them, but respect them the same way you desire respect for yourself.

It's not uncommon for boys or girls at sometime during their early teens to have feelings for someone of the same sex or have an experience (say a group of boys masturbating to see who is most macho) that may make a person wonder if he could be gay. But one isolated experience does not mean a person is gay.

However, if a teen *consistently* finds himself attracted to males rather than females, he is likely homosexual. That is who he is; that is his sexuality. Because heterosexuality is more common than homosexuality, some families have difficulty understanding homosexuality.*

No person, whoever he or she is, should be discriminated against or shunned. We're all equal human beings. I could have easily been born homosexual rather than heterosexual, right-handed rather than left-handed, brown eyed rather than blue, or born to a family with a different skin color or culture. Our differences are what make each of us unique and interesting. What do you think of people who are different from you? I'm usually curious about how they live, what they think, and their values.

Michael, your sexual values emerge from your sexuality, how you feel about yourself, and your body. Your sexuality is directly tied to your self-esteem, how you feel about your whole self.

*For a list of books to help families needing more information on homosexuality see Additional Reading in the back of this book.

Your self-esteem determines your outlook on life and how you get along in the world—the relationships you have with family, friends, and co-workers.

We'll talk more about self-esteem and relationships in my letters on dating. Now you need to become comfortable with your sexuality by studying your body and learning how your reproductive and sexual anatomy works.

You should feel comfortable with your sexuality, Michael. The only time sex isn't healthy is when:

◆ you have sex with someone for your own self-centered pleasure and you don't care about them (use a person for sex)

◆ you have intercourse without birth control and STD protection

◆ you have intercourse before you're emotionally able to handle the intimacy

◆ having sex goes against your religious or moral values

◆ you use sex to hurt, abuse, or dominate another person

◆ you become so obsessed with sex that it dominates your life.

Though there may be certain times in your teens when you think you are obsessed with sex, usually it only seems that way and doesn't require a counselor's attention. But if you become concerned, talk to someone.

At first you may feel modest and self-conscious about your new body. That's normal, and modesty is appropriate in public places and social settings. Most of us feel more comfortable walking down a crowded street with our clothes on rather than off.

When will your body begin to change? It can happen as early as ten or as late as sixteen. The first changes you may notice are the beginning of pubic hair and having wet dreams. The following letters will let you know what body changes to expect so you are prepared to handle the changes.

If, after you read this letter, you want more information on a particular body change or you have other questions ask me or your dad. If we don't know the answers, we'll help you find them.

*Mom,*

*You say I should feel good about myself, but I can count at least three things that really bug me. I wish I was a different height, had a larger chest and shoulders and that I didn't have acne.*

Michael, all of us have things we'd like to change about our appearance, and we often compare ourselves with other people. I have always wanted to be thin and have blond hair like my friend Ginny. But I don't have blond hair, nor will my body ever be twenty pounds thinner.

Your body is only a covering for the you inside. Your personality and smile will make you more successful and win you more friends than any body-building program.

My next few letters illustrate body development and give you information on how to take care of your body. I included pubic hair growth, chest, voice, penis and scrotum development, wet dreams, masturbation, erections, conception, and other information about your body. Keep reading.

Take care,
Mom

_____

_____

_____

_____

_____

_____

_____

_____

# LETTER 4

# Body Talk–Body Hair and Skin Care

Dear Michael,

Young males and females experience hair and skin changes, especially during puberty. This letter tells you what changes to expect and how to take care of yourself through these changes.

## Body Hair

As you go through puberty, hair growth will appear under your arms, on your face, legs, and possibly on your chest— and for some males, their backs. Hair growth may begin as early as age eight or as late as age sixteen. Body hair is part of having an adult body.

The amount of body hair you will have depends on two things: your heredity and your ethnic background. A male whose father and grandfathers have lots of hair probably will also have a good amount of body hair. Other males, whose fathers and grandfathers have little or no hair on their chests, arms and legs, probably won't be very hairy. Looking at our family background, what amount of hair do you think you'll have?

Your race (Asian, African-American, Caucasian, Hispanic, etc.) also determines the general amount of body hair you'll have. The important point to remember is that having or not having body hair doesn't make you any more, or any less, masculine or attractive. Some women like hairless chests; others like hairy chests.

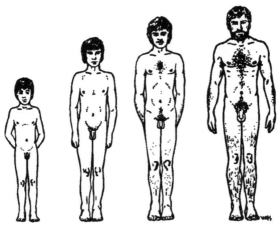

## Male Development

The above illustration shows the four stages of body growth in males.

To understand each change let's break it down. Some of the first body changes males notice are pubic hair and underarm hair growth and skin changes.

Stage 1:
Pubic hair growth begins around the base of the penis as little white bumps or hair follicles. Later, hairs begin growing out of the bumps. If you don't know what's happening, you may wonder if something is wrong, but the growth of hair follicles is how the process starts. You may also notice bumps on the skin of the scrotum and penis that don't grow hair. These are sweat glands. They secrete oil and perspiration.

Stage 2:
Pubic hair continues to grow, becoming curlier, thicker, and darker in color. Pubic hair can be the same color as your hair color or lighter or darker. When people get old their pubic hair is apt to turn gray like the hair on their heads.

Stage 3:
Pubic hair has reached its adult growth pattern. Hair may also grow on your scrotum, around your anus and up towards your navel.

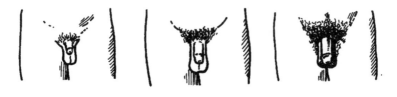

Pubic Hair Growth

## Facial Hair

Sometime during puberty, you will begin to grow hair on your face. Since I don't have any direct experience in this area, I called a local barber school and the following is what they said about facial hair growth, shaving and mustache and beard care.

Facial hair can appear as early as age thirteen, but generally happens around ages fourteen to sixteen. Your first facial hairs will usually start at the outer corners of your lip. Gradually, more hairs will appear inward to form a mustache, although the hair may be light at first and barely visible. Hair will also begin growing on the lower part of your cheeks, on your chin, and along your jawbone. Usually the hair will be light in color and sparse at first, and then grow thicker and darker in color.

You may have full facial hair by age eighteen, or you could be a guy who has little facial hair in your teens or twenties but can grow a full beard and mustache at age thirty. Again, your heredity, in part, determines your facial hair growth.

## Shaving

When should you begin shaving? You should begin shaving when you feel you need to. Some males want to begin shaving at the first signs of facial hair. Some ask their dads, uncles, or grandfathers when they began shaving and use that as a guide. Other guys don't want to hassle with shaving until they have to. Still others won't shave unless they have to because they like the shadow effect or rugged look. It is not true that if you shave early your hair will come back thicker. Age, health, hormones, and heredity, not shaving, determine hair growth.

Fair skinned, blond males may not have to begin shaving as early as other guys, because their blond facial hairs don't show, or they may get facial hair later than their friends. Darker skinned, dark-haired males may get facial hair earlier. For many black males, shaving causes skin problems, and they should delay shaving as long as possible.

Black males and other males with naturally curly, coarse hair may suffer razor bumps from shaving caused by ingrown facial hairs (facial hairs that curl and grow back into the skin). Ingrown hairs can be gently lifted out of the skin (lift, do not pluck) with tweezers.

If a teen male has curly facial hair, it's a good idea to learn proper shaving techniques at an early age and delay shaving as long as possible. A good barber can instruct you on proper skin care and shaving techniques and it's well worth the time and cost. You can ask your dad, uncle, a coach, or other adult male you respect to help you find a barber who will show you the correct shaving methods.

Most guys like to begin shaving with disposable razors and then later try an electric razor to see which type they prefer.

Let me know if you want me to put disposable razors and shaving cream on the grocery list or if you want to buy them yourself.

The number of shaves you get from a disposable or electric razor will depend on your beard growth and the type of hair you have. A fair-haired male may get a dozen or more shaves. A dark-haired male with thick whisker growth may only get five or six shaves with a disposable razor. If you use a disposable razor it should always be smooth, sharp, and free from nicks, rust, or soap build-up.

The key is the comfort level. When you feel the razor start pulling whiskers rather than making a clean cut—you aren't getting a comfortable or close shave and it's time for a new blade, or your electric razor blades need sharpening.

It's important that you clean the hair out of your razor after every shave according manufacturer's instructions. You should use shaving cream with disposable razors. Never use shaving cream with electric razors.

Black males who shave should use shaving gels made for their skin type.

When you begin shaving, you may only have to shave a portion of your face where you have a few hairs. Or you may have to shave both cheeks and your jawline toward your neck.

Hair grows in different directions depending on your personal growth pattern. The direction the blade is pulled across the beard makes a big difference in getting a close shave and this can only be determined by experimentation and experience. At first you may not get a smooth shave, but with practice you'll be able to achieve a close, clean shave. The key to a close, clean shave is to shave into the whisker growth and hold the razor at an angle so it shears the whiskers rather than cuts them. This takes practice, but in time you'll master the technique.

When you shave, shave slowly and smoothly. When you hurry it's easy to cut yourself. When using a disposable razor, rinse off your razor with hot water every several strokes, and keep your razor clean.

Hair growth will determine how often you must shave: once or twice a day, or two or three times a week. If you do nick yourself, you can buy a styptic pencil at the pharmacy to apply to nicks to stop the bleeding. A small piece of toilet tissue will also work—but don't forget to remove the tissue once the bleeding has stopped. Otherwise, you may walk out of the house with toilet paper on your jaw.

## Mustache and Beard Care

Some men like mustaches and beards. They think a beard or mustache looks good on them—and they don't have to shave daily. Other men think they look good clean-shaven (no facial hair). Males may experience the beginning of facial hair growth in their teens, but many males do not have enough growth for a mustache or a beard until their twenties or thirties.

Although most males don't grow beards until after high school, some males with good facial hair growth like mustaches. As a general rule, a teen male shouldn't grow a mustache until his face has established a fairly solid daily growth of facial hair. Otherwise, the mustache may look thin or scraggly. Be patient. Many men can't grow a good mustache until their twenties, and growing a respectable mustache can take as long as six weeks.

Men who wear mustaches or beards need a regular comb and barber scissors (small but long, pointed scissors which can be bought at any pharmacy and most stores). Household scissors don't work very well on beards and mustaches.

Mustache care is relatively easy. Wash your mustache daily when you shower, comb it as you comb the rest of your hair, and trim it with barber scissors whenever it begins to fall below the lip line. When you get your hair cut, your barber or hair stylist can give your mustache regular trims and advise you on care and style.

You've probably seen handle bar mustaches worn by cowboys in the movies. They take a lot of work and care, including mustache wax on the ends to keep the style. Most men prefer a simple mustache that stops at the corners of the mouth.

Beard care is similar to mustache care. Wash your beard daily with shampoo when you shower, comb it as you comb the rest of your hair, and trim it weekly with barber scissors. If the skin under your beard dries out, work conditioner into the skin and rinse. Your barber or hair stylist can give your beard regular trims and advise you on care and style. A full beard may take an adult male up to two months to grow. Growing time for a close-cut beard may be only thirty days. A close-cut beard looks nice but requires upkeep, including shaving with clippers and a guard.

## Skin Changes

Acne is a body change that is bothersome for many teens. During puberty 79% of teens will be affected by skin problems, such as pimples (zits), whiteheads, blackheads, or acne.

Oil glands in your body produce an oily substance called sebum which keeps skin soft and supple. Unfortunately, these oil glands are especially numerous on your face, neck, shoulders, back, and upper chest. During puberty your oil glands work overtime producing more sebum than you need which results in skin blemishes.

A few teens experience little or no problem with pimples, but the majority of teens have minor to major skin problems. Some teens have acne throughout their teenage years, others for only a year or two. A few people have acne in adulthood. If you experience acne, you are not alone. Most of the kids in your class share the same problem. Acne and the degree of its severity also tends to be hereditary. Teens whose parents had acne as teens will most likely also have acne.

The best treatment to minimize acne is good health and hygiene. Get exercise, eat a balanced diet, get plenty of sleep, and practice good skin care. Wash your body's oily areas with a mild soap and water twice a day (morning and night), shampoo your hair frequently, wear clean clothes, and change clothes daily.

Acne may be especially bothersome on the face, neck, and back. Washing with a mild soap on a clean wash cloth, sponge, or facial scrubber may further help clean the oil out of the skin pores.

Special anti-acne soaps and non-prescription acne medications can help and are available at the pharmacy. For serious acne problems, our family doctor or a dermatologist can prescribe special medication.

Guys may think girls won't date them if they have acne. To most girls it's not an issue, they like you for who you are. If you run into a girl who is hung up on looks, she isn't worth your time anyway.

## Cold Sores (Fever Blisters)

Some people (including teens and children) are bothered by cold sores, and cold sores aren't fun. When you're in school, a cold sore on your lip (much like a pimple on your chin) can feel like a huge blotch on your face. You want it to heal as fast as possible.

Cold sores are caused by a type of herpes virus. Some people carry the virus in their bodies all their lives, while other people are not susceptible. The herpes cold sore virus is not the herpes virus that gives people genital herpes. But, the virus is contagious. So if you have a cold sore or know of someone who does, don't exchange drinking glasses, handkerchiefs, eating utensils, or kisses until the cold sore is healed. Once the virus is in your body, cold sores can break out at any time, especially if you're under stress, have a cold, or the flu. Mild cold sores can be treated with over-the-counter medications. For severe cold sores a doctor can prescribe stronger medication like acyclovir.

## Hemorrhoids

One other body irritation that may or may not affect you is hemorrhoids. Most teens don't have hemorrhoids but you may develop them if you're overweight, or you're a body builder.

Hemorrhoids are caused by excessive pressure placed on particular veins in the abdominal cavity. The most common causes of hemorrhoids are constipation, obesity (being overweight), and in women, pregnancy (usually hemorrhoids in pregnant women heal and disappear after the baby is born).

Hemorrhoids are swollen clusters of veins outside and/or inside your anus that may bleed or make your anal area sore after bowel movements. Blood in your stool is the most common sign of hemorrhoids. However, blood in your stool can also be a sign of other serious disorders, so if you ever notice anything unusual, let me know so we can set up a doctor's appointment.

People often joke about hemorrhoids because they're an irritation people aren't comfortable talking about. Having hemorrhoids isn't usually life threatening, but they are uncomfortable and can be painful. Minor irritations can be controlled with hemorrhoidal creme or a warm bath. Major discomfort may require surgery. To help prevent hemorrhoids, eat plenty of fruits and vegetables, exercise and watch your weight. If you lift weights, be careful not to over-train.

## Body Odor

During puberty, your sweat glands become more active, you perspire more, and have a stronger body odor. In many countries body odor is considered natural and is an accepted odor. But in America we generally don't like to smell body odor. To keep body odor to a minimum, you'll want to take daily showers or baths and use either an underarm antiperspirant or underarm deodorant.

Antiperspirants are designed to minimize perspiration. Deodorants cover or mask perspiration odor. Most girls and guys should begin using these products by at least fifth or sixth grade. Wearing cotton clothing can also minimize odor since cotton absorbs sweat better than synthetics.

Here's a recap of basic hygiene.

- Wash oily areas of your body— face, back, and arms— at least twice a day. Over-the-counter medications can help clear up pimples. For problem acne see a dermatologist.

- Wash your hair daily or at least every other day.

- Adult body odor is strong so bathe or shower daily, and use antiperspirant or deodorant.

Here's to feeling confident about yourself.
Mom

_____

_____

_____

_____

_____

_____

# LETTER 5

# Body Talk —Body Growth

Dear Michael,

Height, chest development, voice changes . . . . These are important body changes that males are concerned about. This letter talks about these changes.

## Height

What height will you be when you reach your full adult size? Will you be medium height, taller or shorter? Your height is in part determined by your heredity—the height your dad and I are and the height of your grandparents.

As a child you usually grew about two inches per year. Then sometime during adolescence, you should have a growth spurt in which you may grow as much as three and a half inches or more a year toward your adult height. This growth spurt generally happens around age thirteen or fourteen, but it may happen at a younger or older age.

It's also common for your feet to grow before your height spurt begins. There are also cases where a male will have reached stage four or five in genital development (Letter 6), but he won't have his height spurt till his senior year. Then he may grow five or six inches in one year. Your growth spurt will be determined by your body's timetable for growth.

Males sometimes worry about their height. They worry that if they are too short or too tall they won't get dates. Guys who are extremely tall (unless they are basketball players) often wish they were shorter, while short guys may wish they were taller. Wishing is okay but it won't add inches to your height. You can be a successful, likable person at whatever height you are—short, tall or medium. If people judge you on your height, they aren't the kind of people you need in your life.

## Chest Development

As your body begins changing and you begin your growth spurt, your chest and shoulders will become broader and more developed and your nipples larger and darker in color.

As your chest and nipples are developing you may also experience some soreness around your nipples and maybe a lumpy feeling under or around the nipple. This is normal. It's a reaction to the new hormones your body is making. Some males experience the soreness or lumps more than others.

During puberty a significant number of males also experience some swelling around the nipple area—one nipple or both. This condition, called gynecomastia, will be more noticeable in some males than in others. Guys who experience gynecomastia often worry they may be growing breasts, but this is only a temporary condition. If you have swelling in the chest area, don't worry. The swelling generally disappears in a year to a year and a half. Males who tend to be overweight may have a tendency toward a more fleshy chest, but guys do not develop breasts like women.

## Voice

During puberty your voice will change because your vocal cords and larynx (voice box) are growing and maturing. Your voice becomes lower and deeper because your vocal chords grow longer and thicker, creating a different sound. This change can happen around fourteen or fifteen and sometimes earlier or later.

Some males don't notice the change much. Others notice it if their voices "crack." Cracking usually occurs when you are talking in a normal voice and your voice gets high or squeaky. Normally, cracking doesn't happen often. If you find your voice cracking, it may help to stay calm, take deep breaths, and speak slowly. The good news is cracking only lasts a year or so until your voice settles into its adult intonation.

Body growth, chest development, and voice are important changes for males, but that's only part of the picture. My next letter details the reproductive system including the penis and testes and that's important info too.

Keep Reading,
Mom

_____

_____

_____

_____

_____

_____

_____

_____

# LETTER 6

# Body Talk
# Penis & Reproductive System

Dear Michael,

Your exterior genitals include your penis, glans (head of the penis), meatus (urethral opening), and scrotum (skin sac which houses the testicles). The anus (see p. 32) is not technically considered part of the genitalia. It is a part of the intestinal system and is the same in both females and males. When we have a bowel movement it dispels solid waste from the large intestine.

Your penis and scrotum are small when you are a boy. When you begin puberty, your penis, testicles, and scrotum will begin growing to their adult size. The five stages of penis, testicles, and scrotum growth are illustrated on page 33. See if you can tell what growth stage you are currently in.

Stage 1:
This is the stage from birth through childhood. The penis and scrotum grow a little larger as you grow, but there's not much change in the basic way they look.

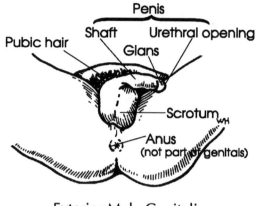

Exterior Male Genitalia

Stage 2:

This stage is the actual beginning of puberty when your testicles begin growing (your penis should begin its growth in Stage 3). As your testicles grow, your scrotal sac begins to hang lower, get wrinkly and baggier, and the skin begins to feel and look different. Dark-skinned males' scrotums will become deeper in color, while fair-skinned males' scrotums take on a reddish tint. Boys usually begin puberty around age twelve, but some boys will begin a year or so earlier or later. This stage may last from five months to twenty-six months, but the average growth period in this stage is about thirteen months.

Stage 3:

By the time you reach stage 3, your penis has begun to grow and you may also notice your first pubic hairs growing around the base of your penis. If you haven't noticed it already, you may see that one testicle also hangs slightly lower than the other. This is normal. Some boys reach stage three at about age thirteen, but others reach it at a younger or older age. Your body's timetable will be right for you. Stage 3 may last from two months to nineteen months, with the average time being about ten months.

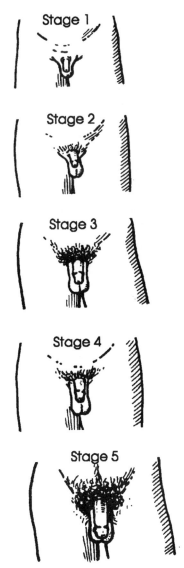

Stage 4:
By the time you reach stage four your penis will have grown quite a bit, both wider and longer, and the head of the penis will be more developed. Boys may reach stage four around age fourteen or a year or more earlier or later. Stage 4 may last five months to three years, with the average time being about two years. This is the longest growth period of the three rapid growth stages.

Stage 5:
This is the last stage of growth and results in the adult penis and scrotum. Some males attain full genital growth around age sixteen, while other guys may reach adult development a year or so earlier or later.

## Penis Size

Guys worry about penis size like girls worry about breast size. They worry that if they don't have a large penis they aren't manly, they won't be able to perform sexually, or no one will want to date them. The truth is penis size has nothing to do with masculinity, sexual pleasure, or performance.

Penis size varies like female breast size varies. The average adult male penis is three to five inches long when flaccid (limp/empty) and five to seven inches long when erect (hard/full). A smaller penis usually gains more inches than a larger penis when erect, so two different size penises when limp, can measure the same size when hard.

Females do not use penis size to determine who they want to date. If a girl is dating you for your body rather than you as a person, she doesn't deserve to date you. Good relationships are based on respect and love, not body parts.

All this information may not be comforting when you are in the locker room and guys are making jokes. One reason some guys tease others is that they are anxious, uncomfortable, or insecure about their own body development. The other reason is that some guys are jerks.

## Circumcision

Male babies are born with a sheath of skin (foreskin) covering the head of the penis. Circumcision is a process where the foreskin covering the glans is cut away. The operation dates back to biblical days and was originally performed as a religious custom. Throughout the generations circumcision has fallen in and out of social favor.

Before the 1940s many males in America were not circumcised. But then the medical community begin urging circumcision for hygienic reasons. Doctors felt that circumcised penises were easier to keep clean and free from disease.

Today circumcision is a choice left up to the parents. Many parents still have their sons circumcised, while other parents elect not to circumcise. Circumcision is usually done in the hospital within a day or so after a baby boy is born. However, some religions adhere to a religious custom where the procedure is performed in a ceremony at home.

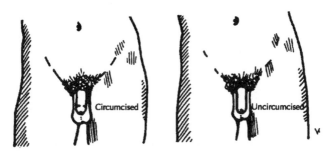

## Circumcised and Uncircumcised Penis

Circumcision is painful for the newborn and some people don't believe it's a necessary operation. If circumcision is not performed as a baby, a boy may elect to be circumcised at an older age—but not many do. In rare cases the foreskin on an uncircumcised male can become tight or stuck to the head of the penis and a circumcision may be necessary to relieve pain or discomfort.

To clean an uncircumcised penis, the foreskin must be pulled back as shown in the illustration below and the inside area gently washed. If the uncircumcised penis is not washed daily, a secretion called smegma collects under the foreskin and causes irritation and odor.

Although circumcised and uncircumcised penises look different, they work the same way. When an uncircumcised male has an erection, the foreskin automatically pulls back a bit from the head of the penis and it looks similar to a circumcised penis.

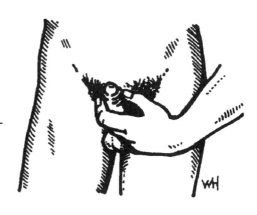

## Washing Uncircumcised Penis

Other than some people feeling that the circumcised penis is easier to keep clean, there are no other advantages or disadvantages of one form over the other.

## Interior Male Reproductive System

While changes are happening outside your body, there are also changes going on inside your reproductive organs. Your interior reproductive anatomy includes the testicles (or testes), vas deferens, ampulla, prostate gland, epididymis, and urethra. Don't let the names scare you, I'll explain them.

### Testicles and Sperm

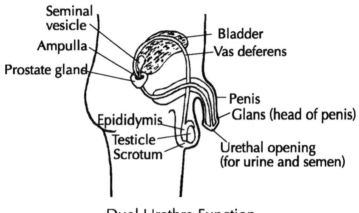

Dual Urethra Function

Your testicles are glands where sperm are made. Sperm is one of the two cells needed to create a baby; the other being the ova from the female body. Males are normally born with two testicles. In rare cases a boy may be born with only one testicle, or sometimes an injury will damage a testicle so it must be removed. Even if a male only has one testicle, he can father children. And having only one testicle does not affect a man's sex life.

Your testicles (testes, balls) are encased in your scrotum that hangs outside your body. People often refer to the scrotum as "balls" because the scrotum encases the oval, ball-shaped testicles. In actuality, your scrotum is your scrotum and your testicles (balls) are housed inside the scrotum.

Your scrotum hangs outside your body because for sperm to be produced, they must have a constant temperature slightly lower than your normal body temperature. If you have a fever, it's hot outside, or you take a hot bath, your scrotum will hang even farther away from your body than usual. Likewise in cold weather or if you jump into a cold pool, your scrotum brings your testicles closer to your body for warmth.

Before you are born your testicles are inside your body just under your penis. When you are born they come down (descend) into the scrotal sac. Once in a while, only one testicle descends, and the other is undescended. No one knows for sure what causes an undescended testicle but doctors can perform surgery to bring it down.

Your testicles are actually made up of hundreds of tiny compartments and inside these compartments are tubules, tiny thread-like tubes all coiled together. It is here that sperm is made. You will begin making sperm at the onset of puberty (somewhere between nine and fourteen years of age) and keep making new sperm every day until you are in your sixties or older.

Sperm are living cells that look like tadpoles, but they are so small that during intercourse in one ejaculation (release of semen from the penis) millions of sperm are deposited in the female

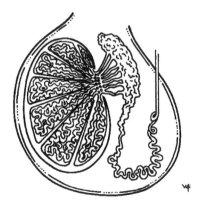

Cross Section of Scrotum

vagina. In part, that's why it is so easy for a guy to get a girl pregnant. It only takes one sperm from the millions you ejaculate to find the girl's ovum and fertilize it—and sperm are tough, fast, swimmers.

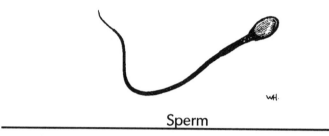

---
#### Sperm
---

## Epididymis

After sperm are made in your testicles, they travel to your epididymis (the storage compartment and passageway from the testicles to the vas deferens) where they are stored for about six weeks to achieve maturity. You can feel your epididymis (and vas deferens) as a raised section on the back of your testicle.

## Vas Deferens and Ampulla

Once they have developed to maturity, your sperm can then survive at body temperature and travel upward through your vas deferens (sperm ducts) to the ampulla. The ampulla is the storage compartment where sperm are stored to await mixing with the semen for ejaculation. You have two sperm ducts (tubes), one for each testicle, but in the illustration on page 36 you can only see one of them.

## Seminal Vesicles and Prostate Gland

Attached to your ampulla are two seminal vesicles, one for each of your sperm ducts. Your seminal vesicles produce semen, the milky white fluid that mixes with the sperm for ejaculation.

Semen (slang names: cum or jism) is full of protein and sugars providing the sperm with the energy needed once they are ejaculated into a female's vagina to swim all the way to her fallopian tubes, find the ova, and unite with it.

Your prostate gland lies below your ampulla. During ejaculation it puts pressure on your vas deferens to push the semen into your urethra—while the ampulla adds fluid to the semen.

## Urethra

The inside of your penis is made of spongy tissue. The urethra is a hollow tube that runs down the middle of the penis to the glans (tip of the penis). The urethra is connected to your bladder and your vas deferens—one of the places your sperm are stored. The urethra is unique because it releases both urine (slang: pee, piss) and sperm—but never at the same time.

The idea of the urethra releasing both urine and sperm may at first seem gross, but nature has it all figured out. Your urine and semen *never mix*. Before you ejaculate (release semen), a special valve on your bladder automatically shuts off all urine flow, to allow the flow of semen. Glands in that area then release a tiny amount of liquid into the urethra to flush it clean before the semen flows through. We'll talk about ejaculation in detail later in this letter.

Although some people are susceptible to urinary and intestinal infections, in general your bladder and intestines should function smoothly. To help prevent potential problems, always practice good hygiene.

## Genital Care and Hygiene

* Wash your penis, scrotal area, and anus daily when you shower or bathe.

* Always try to avoid direct hits to your penis and scrotum. A direct hit can render you unconscious. A severe injury could damage your ability to make sperm.

  Baseball and high-contact sports like kick-boxing require that you wear a jock strap (cloth supporter) with a plastic cup inside to protect your penis and testes from injury. You can also wear a jock strap without a cup, for light contact sports, but some males feel their jockey shorts give them enough support without a jock strap. It's really a matter of personal comfort or what the coach advises. Jock straps come in small, medium, and large sizes according to your waist size. Cups come in sizes too, which can vary from small youth to large adult.

* Accidents can happen. Anytime you get hit in the penis or scrotum, if the pain doesn't go away after a few minutes, immediately put an ice pack on the injury. If the ice doesn't help and you still have pain and or swelling a few hours later, let someone look at it, go see a doctor, or go to a hospital emergency room. You need medical care.

* Wear all-cotton underwear. Synthetics can cause irritation by trapping bacteria in the genital area. Cotton lets your body breathe.

* Don't wear extremely tight underwear or exercise shorts for long periods of time, because tight clothing can cause skin irritations like jock itch (a fungus infection that causes itching and soreness of your genitals and inner thighs).

* If you are prone to jock itch (slang: jock rot), rubbing cornstarch on the area may help cure the problem or you can buy non-prescription creams and sprays. Occasionally a doctor will need to prescribe a medicine, but keeping the irritated area dry and clean, avoiding tight clothing, and wearing clean clothes can do much to prevent or cure the problem.

* If you ever have pain when urinating or having a bowel movement or if you ever notice blood in your urine or your stools, tell me immediately so we can have it checked out. As a young adult, blood in your stools can be something as simple as hemorrhoids, and pain when urinating can be a simple urinary infection; but any health concern should always be checked out by a doctor. Genital irritations should be cleared up as quickly as possible so they won't turn into a serious problem. It's important to keep your body healthy.

* Once you begin making sperm and experience your first wet dream or ejaculation, you need to begin a monthly testicle self-exam.

## Testicular Self-exams (TSE) Help Detect Cancer

The testicle self-exam consists of observing your testicles once a month for any odd lumps or bumps—which might be cancer or other medical problem.

Once a month, after a shower or hot bath when your scrotum is most relaxed you should perform a testicle self-exam. Gently examine each testicle by putting your thumb on the top of your testicle and your index and middle fingers on the underside of your testicle. Now roll your testicle gently between your thumb and finger, feeling for any small lump—pea size or larger. Any abnormality will most often be felt as a firm area on the side or front of the testicle. The epididymis on the back of your testicle may feel different than the rest of your testicle, but that's normal.

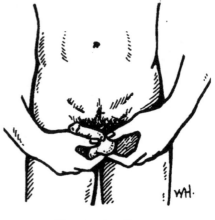

Testicular Exam

Although testicular cancer accounts for less than 1% of all cancers, it is the most common cancer for men ages twenty to thirty-five years (and for men whose testicles descended after age six or men whose testicles never descended into the scrotum).

Most men diagnosed with testicular cancer first discover it by self-exam. If you begin self-exams in your teens, they should become a routine you perform each month, especially during the high risk years (ages twenty to thirty-five).

Most lumps on the scrotum are not cancer, but cysts. Cysts are collections of fluid and most will go away by themselves. Others may require surgery to be removed.

For sports physicals or any complete physical, the doctor usually performs a testicular exam. He may then give you TSE information to take home so you can begin performing the exam yourself.

Sometimes males are uncomfortable the first time they go for a sports physical because they have heard friends talk about the exam. Your dad said that when he had his first sports physical, the upperclassmen on the team told him the doctor was going to hold his balls to perform a testicular exam and make him cough to check for abnormal lumps or masses. That's what the doctor did.

Your dad said he has one word for you about testicular exams—*relax*. It only takes a few seconds, and it's an important test, and many doctors today perform the exam without asking the patient to cough.

## Other Medical Conditions

### Twisted testicles

Twisted testicles are rare, but if they do occur, immediate surgery is required. Twisted testicles usually occur following some type of physical exertion. No one knows why they happen, but they cause extreme pain, nausea, vomiting, and fever. If you or a friend ever have these symptoms during or after sports or other physical activity, get medical help immediately, even if you have to dial 911.

### Swollen glands

The genital area contains lymph glands which can occasionally become infected. This causes pain and swelling, but can usually be cured with antibiotics.

### Aching balls (blue balls)

This isn't a problem requiring medical help, but it can cause pain in the testicles or genital area. This discomfort occurs when a male has an erection for a long time without ejaculating. A kissing or making-out session where you've had an erection for a long time can cause this aching, and even after the erection subsides, the pain may continue. This is because the blood was trapped in the penis for a long time. Although it is uncomfortable, the pain goes away in a few hours.

## Hernias

Another condition that males need to watch for is the hernia. Hernias can happen to females too, but men who lift heavy objects in their work or at home are more apt to develop hernias. A hernia occurs when part of the intestines bulge through a weak spot in the abdominal wall. The weakness is usually corrected through surgery. If this happens in the lower abdomen, it can cause genital pain.

Symptoms of a hernia include a soft lump or swelling on the top or side of the scrotum or in the crease where the thigh and groin meet. If you ever experience sudden pain in the groin along with nausea, it could be a strangulated hernia that needs immediate surgery. Go to the hospital emergency room or see a doctor immediately.

## Prostate trouble

As males age, the prostate gland expands exerting pressure on the urethra, making it more difficult to urinate completely (empty your bladder). Males generally don't have to worry about this until their sixties or seventies. The prostate gland is also a common site for cancer in older men. For this reason, doctors have recommended annual exams for prostate problems beginning at age forty.

Rectal exams used to be the standard procedure for detection. Now there is a blood test that tests for prostate cancer. This test may be ordered in place of or in conjunction with a rectal exam. Like a testicular exam, the rectal exam only lasts a few seconds.

You've learned about the different parts of your reproductive system and how they work, and about common injuries and medical problems. The next letter on your urinary and intestinal system is also important.

Take care,
Mom

_____

_____

_____

_____

_____

_____

_____

_____

_____

_____

# LETTER 7

# Body Talk—Urinary and Intestinal Systems

Dear Michael,

As you are beginning to see, your body is a complicated machine with many interrelated parts. While the urinary and intestinal systems are not part of your reproductive system, they perform important bodily functions, and you need to understand how they work and how to care for them.

Anatomically, your intestinal system actually starts with your mouth and includes your esophagus, stomach, large and small intestines, rectum, and anus. For now, we're only concerned with the abdominal area. Your large intestines (bowels) break down solid wastes from your stomach into feces (slang: poop) which is expelled down your rectum and out your anus.

Your urinary system begins with the bladder collecting and breaking down liquid wastes and expelling them as urine (slang: pee) through the urethra. In males the urethra expels both urine and semen but never at the same time.

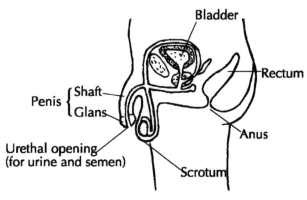

## Urinary and Intestinal System

Although some people are susceptible to urinary and intestinal infections, the bladder and intestines usually function smoothly. Good hygiene can help prevent problems.

* Wash your penis and anus daily when you shower or bathe. If you are uncircumcised, pull the foreskin back and wash the underside daily (see illustration on page 35).

* Wear all-cotton underwear. Synthetics can cause irritation by trapping bacteria in the genital area. Cotton lets your body breathe.

* Anytime you notice blood in your stools or pain when urinating or during a bowel movement, tell me immediately so we can have it checked out.

* Irritations should be cleared up as quickly as possible so they don't turn into problem infections.

My next letter is about erections, wet dreams and masturbation.

Keep Reading,
Mom

_____
_____
_____

# Letter 8

# Body Talk—Erections, Wet Dreams and Masturbation

Dear Michael,

You may be thinking, "Mom is talking to me about wet dreams, masturbation, and erections. This is too embarrassing!"

Michael, these occurrences are all normal activities for males, and you need to know what to expect. Although people don't generally talk about these topics at the dinner table, erections, wet dreams, and masturbation are a normal part of becoming a man.

## Erections

Your penis can be soft and flaccid (empty) or hard and erect (full). During an erection (slang: hard on, boner) blood fills the spongy tissue of your penis and the muscles at the base of your penis tighten so the blood stays in the penis. This makes your penis harder, longer, and thicker. It may stick upward or outward from your body. Erect penises can be straight or slightly curved, stiff and hard, or semi-hard, and each variation is normal.

49

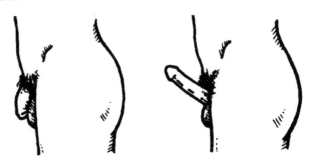

### Flaccid and Erect Penis

Males can have erections for various reasons and at various times. You can have an erection if your penis is rubbed or touched, you're thinking sexual thoughts, you're nervous or excited, you're having warm-hearted thoughts, and even if your penis hasn't been touched and you aren't thinking about anything in particular. You can also have an erection waking up from sleeping. Often this isn't a true erection, but your penis becomes larger because you have a full bladder and need to urinate. For males, an erection is a normal body function.

After you have an erection, your penis will then return to its soft, empty state in one of two ways:

- Your erection will eventually subside by itself. This may take a few seconds, a couple of minutes, or several minutes. Your muscles can't stay tightened forever, so eventually your muscles relax, the blood flows back out of the spongy tissue in the penis, and your penis returns to its flaccid (limp) state.

- Your erection may also subside by ejaculation through masturbation, nocturnal emission (wet dream), or intercourse—and we'll talk about all of these activities in detail later.

## Spontaneous Erections

Males can have erections from birth, onward, but most males find that once they begin puberty, they have erections more frequently than before. Some of these erections are spontaneous —erections that happen at anytime, anywhere, for no particular or specific reason. Spontaneous erections can happen anytime, anywhere—at school, home, playing sports. As one teen told me, guys feel as self-conscious about these types of erections as girls feel about getting their periods during school. Here's one guy's story.

> I'm a jock. I play basketball, football, and run track. When my body started changing I tried to act cool, but I was actually very self-conscious. One day I was walking down the hall in school and had an erection. I thought, 'What do I do now? I'm not even thinking about sex, but everyone is going to notice this bulge in my jeans.' All I can remember is that I took my books and carried them in front of me, praying that the erection would go away fast.

Once you reach puberty you can also have erections simply by looking at a female or thinking about sex. The best way to deal with an erection at home, school, in a public place, or on a date is to pretend nothing is happening. Continue with what you're doing, breathe slowly, think non-sexual thoughts, and relax. When you're wearing jeans, most people won't even notice your erection, and even if someone does notice, they should also ignore it.

The first time you have an erection in public can be embarrassing, but remember, most people won't even notice—and all males your age are experiencing the same trials of growing up. You may want to ask your dad or uncle if they ever had an embarrassing situation with an erection. Later on, if you date, simple kissing or making-out will trigger an erection.

## Ejaculation

Ejaculation is the release of semen down the urethra and out of the penis. Your genital muscles, helped by your prostate gland, contract or tighten and the continual contractions (tightening) force the semen down the urethra and out the meatus (urethral opening in the end of your penis).

Remember that the valve on your bladder has shut off urine flow to allow you to ejaculate semen. The semen, usually a teaspoon or two of white, creamy liquid, normally comes out of the penis in three or four spurts. Many boys experience their first ejaculation around age twelve or thirteen, but some don't ejaculate until they are fifteen or older. Your first ejaculation usually occurs through masturbation or a wet dream.

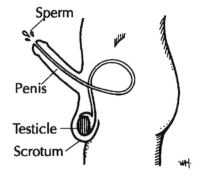

Ejaculation Process

## Orgasm

The pleasurable, tingly feeling you have when the nerve endings in your penis contract to a point of release is called an orgasm (slang: climax, coming, getting off). Orgasm is a normal, healthy sensory response. Males usually experience orgasm by masturbation, wet dreams, oral stimulation, or intercourse. Females also experience orgasm, by manual or oral stimulation of the clitoris or by friction on the clitoris during intercourse.

Once males begin puberty, they usually ejaculate and reach orgasm at the same time. As a child, you can have orgasms when you masturbate, but you don't ejaculate until you begin making sperm during puberty.

## Wet Dreams

An experience of puberty that most guys feel a little uneasy about is nocturnal (night) ejaculations or "wet dreams." The wet dream is so named because it happens when you are sleeping and is usually accompanied by sexual dreams. While sleeping or dreaming you get an erection and ejaculate. It's normal for boys during puberty to have sexual dreams—sometimes very vivid dreams. That doesn't mean you are oversexed, it's just your body's way of dealing with puberty. Other times, you may have wet dreams (ejaculate) even though you don't recall dreaming. You will probably have wet dreams more frequently during puberty than any other time in your life.

During puberty your hormones are working so hard your body makes an excess supply of sperm. One of the ways your body rids itself of that sperm is through a wet dream. When you awaken, you'll find one to two tablespoons of semen on your belly, pajamas or your sheets. Wet dreams can begin as early as age ten or as late as age fourteen. A guy's first wet dream can be as much a surprise to him as having a period is to a girl.

Wet dreams are nothing to worry about. They are a normal part of growing up. Put your pajamas/sheets in the laundry as you normally would and go on with your day. Wet dreams happen to almost every male during puberty. The good news is that after you finish puberty wet dreams don't happen often.

## Masturbation

Masturbation or self-pleasuring is stroking or rubbing the penis to produce ejaculation or orgasm. A male most often uses one hand to massage the penis; a female uses her fingers to massage the clitoris. Many boys and girls discover masturbation as babies or small children but forget about it until puberty. Having sexual thoughts or fantasies when you masturbate is also normal. You are normal if you do or if you don't masturbate.

In earlier times people didn't understand masturbation. It was believed if you masturbated you would go blind or crazy, grow hair on your palms, get warts or pimples, or use up all of your sperm. It was feared that males would damage their penises and that females would hurt themselves so they couldn't have children. If you masturbated before a sports event you would hurt your playing ability. Today we know these are all just superstitions.

Some of the slang terms for masturbation include jacking off, jerking off, beating your meat, and playing with yourself. People use these rude slang terms because they are uncomfortable talking about masturbation. This can be especially true of teens who are not yet comfortable with their sexuality. They may accuse others of jerking off because they are not comfortable admitting to themselves that they also masturbate.

Although self-touching is not something that people talk about at the dinner table, surveys show that most people masturbate. Masturbation is a private activity.

You may have heard the myths that masturbating means you are gay, or if you masturbate that means you're not "getting" any (having sex). These are just myths. You are not gay if you masturbate, and people masturbate whether they are or aren't having sex. For a teen couple, self or partner stimulation is much safer than having sex and risking becoming teen parents.

Masturbation is a natural, healthy way to release sexual tension when you are sexually aroused (slang: turned-on, horny). It is also a private way for you to become comfortable with your body and your sexuality. Masturbation isn't just for teens who aren't having sex. People masturbate throughout their lives.

Males often masturbate more frequently during puberty. Your body is making so much sperm you may feel almost jittery. Releasing built-up sperm through masturbation helps you relax. A male may masturbate once or twice a week, once a day, twice a day, or sometimes several times a day. Males who don't feel comfortable masturbating often have more wet dreams because the semen build up needs to be released.

Some boys have their first masturbation experience by masturbating in a group or with a friend. This is also normal—and it doesn't mean you are gay if you've masturbated with someone.

When teen males masturbate (or have wet dreams) they are sometimes embarrassed about the semen on their pajamas, underwear or bed sheets. There's nothing to be embarrassed about, just throw your clothes in the wash and they'll get washed. Your dad and your uncles had the same problem when they were teens.

If you masturbate do not put your hand over your urethral opening to stop the semen flow. This can result in the semen backing up in your urethra and emptying into the tube coming from your bladder. This situation, called retrograde ejaculation, can cause pain in your penis and genital area, a discharge from your penis, and sometimes a bladder or urinary infection. Also, if you don't like the stickiness on your clothes, you can wipe the semen off your clothes or sheets afterwards with a dry washcloth, or catch the semen in a tissue and throw the tissue in the trash.

## Intercourse

Intercourse, insertion of the male penis into the female vagina, is the third way to release sperm build up. But there are many decisions you have to make before adding sexual intercourse to a relationship.

A young man must guard against getting a girl pregnant, contracting sexually-transmitted diseases (STDs), and both partners must agree to have sex. No one, male or female, has the right to force someone to have sex. Forcing someone to have sex is rape. Rape is a serious crime and we'll talk about that in my letter on sexual abuse.

Until you are in a long-term committed relationship and ready to handle the birth control and STD responsibilities of having sex, the safest way to release sperm build up is through masturbation or wet dreams.

Because of the emotional and practical aspects of having sex, such as birth control and STD responsibilities, young people should be in, at least, their late teens (age eighteen or nineteen) or older and in a long-term committed relationship before having sex. I'll talk about having sex in more detail in later letters.

My next letter is about conception and pregnancy and the man's role in helping his partner through pregnancy. This is information every male needs to know so keep reading.

Take care,
Mom

_____

_____

_____

_____

_____

_____

_____

_____

# LETTER 9

# CONCEPTION AND PREGNANCY— THE MALE'S ROLE

Dear Michael,

Parents and teens often find the topics of conception and pregnancy the most difficult to discuss. In some cases, parents may not know the correct information because their parents never knew or communicated it to them. I hope this letter gives you a solid understanding of the subject.

As you may know from health class, human conception—the creation of new life—normally happens through intercourse.

Pre-teens often find the idea of intercourse gross. They wonder if their parents still "do it." If two people are relaxed and feel comfortable with each other, intercourse can be a pleasurable, loving activity they can enjoy even into their seventies, eighties, and nineties.

When a female wants to have intercourse and she is relaxed and comfortable, her vagina will secrete a small amount of fluid on its walls so the penis can slide into the vagina. Usually the vagina lubricates itself when the female is sexually aroused (slang: turned-on, horny) during foreplay (kissing, and touching body parts before intercourse).

If the vagina has self-lubricated it will easily accommodate the penis, and intercourse is pleasant for both the male and female. Intercourse can be painful for both the man and woman if the female is not ready for intercourse and the vagina is not lubricated. You may wonder how intercourse works. Below is an illustration of the erect penis inside the vagina.

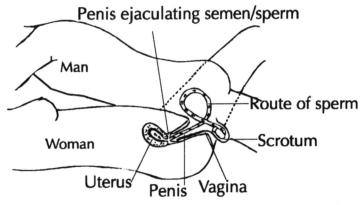

Intercourse should only happen when two people mutually agree to have sex (forced intercourse is rape—a serious crime). To have intercourse the male's penis becomes erect (hard), and he inserts it into the female's vagina. When ejaculation occurs, semen and sperm are released into the vagina.

Sperm are so small that more than three million sperm can be released into the vagina in one ejaculation, and it takes only *one* sperm to make a girl pregnant. Unless you are planning a family, you should never have sex without birth control—just imagine the 3,000,000 sperm in each ejaculation swimming toward the one ovum.

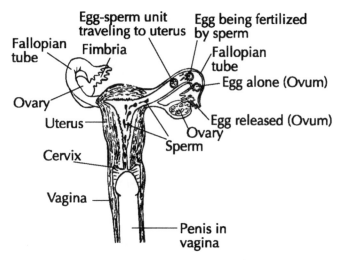

Egg-sperm unit traveling to uterus
Egg being fertilized by sperm
Fallopian tube
Fimbria
Fallopian tube
Egg alone (Ovum)
Ovary
Uterus
Egg released (Ovum)
Ovary
Cervix
Sperm
Vagina
Penis in vagina

## Sperm's Trip From Penis to Fertilize Ovum

After ejaculation, sperm in the semen immediately begin swimming toward the top of the vagina, through the cervix and uterus, and into the fallopian tubes looking for an ovum (egg cell) to fertilize. If they don't find an ovum, they die. Sperm that don't make it to the fallopian tubes fall back into the semen which trickles down the vagina and out of the woman's body. They too die.

Sperm can live in the uterus and fallopian tubes up to three days before dying making it easy for the girl to become pregnant.

After conception (the beginning of pregnancy) the fertilized ovum (zygote) travels down the fallopian tube into the uterus where it attaches itself to the uterine wall. Once attached and allowed to develop, it will grow into a baby.

Occasionally the body naturally aborts (miscarries) the pregnancy. Doctors suspect miscarriages occur because the fertilized ovum was defective in some way, or the woman's body was not ready to sustain the pregnancy.

In a fertilized ovum there are twenty-three pairs of chromosomes plus one X and one X or Y chromosome, representing the exact blueprint of how we will develop—our hair color, height, weight. . .everything. It's a miracle how one ovum and one sperm, when united, can in nine months become a wailing eight pound little person.

## Fathering a Child

Without using birth control and using it correctly, a girl can become pregnant any time she has sex, including the first time. The only 100% effective method of you not getting someone pregnant is abstinence—not having sex, postponing sex until you are in a long-term committed relationship. If you do not choose abstinence, you will need to use some other highly effective birth control method.

Birth control is both *the man and woman's responsibility*. Unless researchers come up with a male pill, the best birth control method for men is the pre-lubricated condom. Pre-lubricated condoms contain nonoxyl 9, which kills the ejaculated sperm. You can read about condoms and how to put them on correctly in Letter 19 on birth control.

When the time comes that you begin having intercourse, unless you are married, you must use a condom every time to protect yourself from contracting a sexually-transmitted diseases or getting someone pregnant.

Even if the girl is on the pill or Norplant®, use a pre-lubricated condom. Young women get pregnant on the pill because they don't take it correctly. Also antibiotics and other drugs may interfere with its effectiveness. If the girl doesn't want you to use a condom, you have to tell her no condom, no sex.

If you are married and an unplanned pregnancy occurs, you and your wife have a more solid ground for handling parenthood. If you are a teen and an unplanned pregnancy happens, you and your girlfriend's lives are changed forever.

Once you are married, and your wife chooses to go on the pill or use the diaphragm, or other effective contraceptive, you may decide as a couple that you don't need additional condom protection.

I hope you won't have sex until you find a person with whom you want a long-term, committed relationship. Most people don't find those relationships until after high school.

One of the reasons so many teens become teen parents is that they add sex to their relationships too early, and they don't use birth control or don't use it correctly. If a couple can't talk openly about birth control and use it correctly, they aren't ready to have sex. Being a teen father severely limits your school activities, your time with friends, and your future plans.

## Pregnancy

The first signs that a female is pregnant are usually nausea (an upset stomach), vomiting, tender breasts, and most importantly, a missed period. Anytime a female thinks she may be pregnant she can take a home pregnancy test or see a doctor to determine if she is pregnant. If a young woman chooses to keep the pregnancy she needs immediate pre-natal medical care.

A full-term pregnancy is approximately 280 days long (forty weeks or nine full lunar months). After the first forty-eight hours the developing fertilized ovum is called a zygote. After fourteen days the zygote is called an embryo, and it has, by then, attached itself to the uterus. At eight weeks human features become apparent and the developing life is called a fetus. The fetus develops into a baby.

During the first three months (first trimester) of pregnancy, most women experience what is called morning sickness— anything from a mildly upset stomach to vomiting. This is the body's reaction to the changes going on inside. I had morning sickness during my pregnancy with you and your sister.

During the *first trimester* pregnant women usually are more tired and may go to bed earlier or need an extra nap after work and on weekends. Being tired is normal as your wife's body adjusts to all the new changes going on in her body to carry the pregnancy.

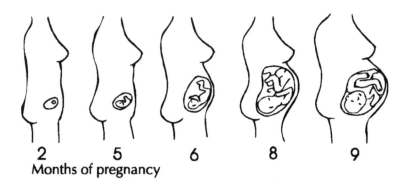

2      5      6      8      9
Months of pregnancy

## Fetal Development Inside Mother

To assure proper pre-natal care, your wife needs to visit the doctor monthly. It's also vital that neither she nor you smoke. Her own smoking, or second-hand smoke from you, is inhaled into her lungs, directly affecting development of the baby. Drinking alcohol, taking drugs, and even too much caffeine are harmful, also. Smoking, alcohol, drugs, and caffeine can severely affect the baby's development and cause birth defects.

Throughout the pregnancy your wife will need your help, and you will need each other for support. Make sure she gets the extra sleep she needs. Help the house run smoothly by doing more of the household chores. If your wife has a normal pregnancy without complications, and she works outside the home, she should be able to continue working until she delivers. But she does need more sleep and she will appreciate the extra help around the house.

During pregnancy, it's common for both partners to feel a little nervous. "Am I sure I'm ready for parenthood?" "Can we be good parents?" The best thing to do is to talk over your fears with each other and reassure each other throughout the pregnancy.

During the *second three months* of pregnancy, (the second trimester) a woman usually regains energy and feels the best she'll feel throughout the pregnancy. Her abdominal area will begin to grow outward (she'll begin to show) as the uterus and fetus are growing.

Toward the middle or end of the second trimester, you may be able to put your hand on your wife's stomach and feel your baby kicking. Babies can also hear inside the uterus so you can talk to your baby to get it used to hearing you and your wife's voices. Your Dad and I talked and sang to you and your sister when you were in the uterus. I felt good the second trimester; but the third trimester was not so easy.

In the *last trimester*, a woman's wrists and joints swell from extra body fluid and her internal organs are all compressed and out of position to make room for the baby. Carrying the baby is exhausting. She often feels heavy, sluggish and unattractive.

When she looks down, her belly is so full of baby she can't see her feet—she wonders if the delivery date will ever arrive.

Imagine if you were to get a teen girl pregnant, and she had to deal with the strain a pregnancy puts on her body? What do you think it would be like if men gave birth instead of women?

Pregnancy is an adult undertaking that demands support by the father of the child to his pregnant partner. Having a baby is the greatest experience in the world—but only if the couple is ready to be parents.

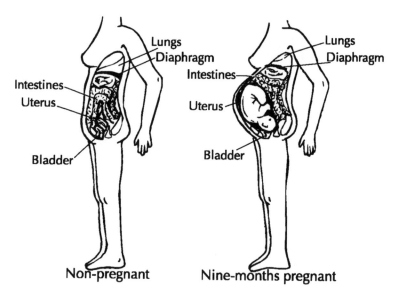

Lungs
Diaphragm
Intestines
Lungs
Diaphragm
Intestines
Uterus
Uterus
Bladder
Bladder
Non-pregnant          Nine-months pregnant

**Female's Internal Organ Placement**

## Childbirth

Childbirth is hard work for the mother, the baby, and the father. At the end of the ninth month, when the baby is ready to be born, the woman's uterus begins to contract. She begins having regular muscle cramps and is said to be "in labor." Scientists don't understand exactly how the female body knows when to begin labor, but labor has its own schedule. During labor the uterine muscles build strength and the cervix and vagina dilate (widen) so the baby can be pushed through the vagina into the world.

During childbirth you can greatly help your wife by talking to her, holding her hand, rubbing her back, helping her breath, counting through the contractions—and just being

# Letter 10

# What You Should Know About Girls' Bodies

Dear Michael,

While you are developing and changing, so are the girls in your class. Your dad told me that at age fourteen, he found one of his uncle's *Playboy* magazines and spent hours wondering what teachers and girls in his class looked like without clothes. When I was in junior high, I wanted to know if penises were different sizes and how jock straps worked. It's perfectly natural for males and females to be curious about each others' bodies.

Because a girl becomes pregnant through intercourse, it's essential that you know how the female body works. During puberty females also experience body changes and body growth.

This letter will explain those changes in detail so you will know exactly how a girl's body works and the body care she needs to keep healthy.

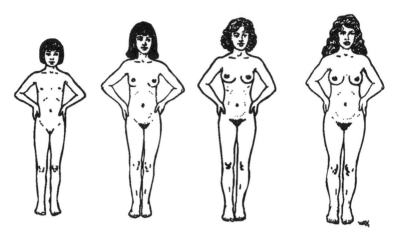

## Female Development From Girl to Woman

## Breasts

One of the first things guys usually notice about girls are their breasts. Boobs, titties, watermelons, knockers— throughout history males have created many slang names for breasts, because men like female breasts. Your dad says he likes breasts because they are warm, soft, and sexy.

Females experience five stages of breast development (p. 71). A girl's body may begin changing as early as age ten or as late as age sixteen.

### The mature female breast

Although you can only see three lobes in the illustration on page 72, the female breast is made up of fifteen to twenty-five lobes all packed together in a circle surrounding the areola and nipple. The inside of the breast lobes are tree-like. The alveoli, the tree's leaves, are where milk is made. Breasts only make milk when a woman has a baby. Milk production does not depend upon breast size.

## The Five Stages of Breast Development

**Stage 1:**
Childhood breasts are flat. The only raised part is the nipple.

**Stage 2:**
Breast-bud stage. Milk ducts and fat tissue grow larger; the areolas widen and become darker in color.

**Stage 3:**
Breasts become more round and full and begin to stand out more. Breasts are often cone-shaped at this stage and that's normal.

**Stage 4:**
In this stage the areola and nipple form a separate mound that protrudes above the breast. Some girls do not go through this stage, and thus their areolas and nipple area does not stand out.

**Stage 5:**
The mature breast is fully developed as determined by the female's genetic, family heredity. Mature breasts come in all sizes—round, full, slender, small, medium, larger, and cone-shaped.

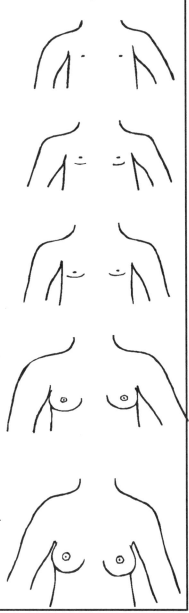

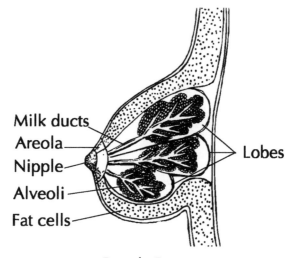

Milk ducts
Areola
Nipple
Alveoli
Fat cells
Lobes

### Female Breast

Female breast size is genetic (dependent upon the breast size of females on both sides of the family tree). Some girls have small breasts, others large breasts. Despite what advertising would like us to think, large breasts are not better than small breasts. In fact, today, extremely large-breasted women sometimes have their breasts surgically reduced because the weight of their breasts is tiring, uncomfortable, and can cause back problems.

### Breast care

It is important that girls take care of their breasts. Until a girl begins menstruating, all she needs to do is wash her breasts daily with the rest of her body, decide if and when she wants to begin wearing a bra, and buy bras that fit comfortably.

After she begins menstruating (gets her period), she should start performing a monthly breast self-exam. A breast self-exam allows a girl to examine her breasts for any lumps or irregularities that might be signs of cancer. If a girl finds anything abnormal, including a nipple suddenly inverting or protruding, she should see a doctor. Cancer is rare in young women, but there are non-cancerous conditions that can affect the breast. If any abnormality lasts more than two weeks, she needs to see a doctor.

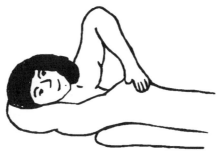

Breast Self-exam

The good news is that breast cancer in teens is very rare, and many lumps that women find in their breasts are *not* cancerous. However, women who have a history of breast cancer in their families should be especially watchful from their teen years on. Even Grandmas should do monthly exams, as well as have a yearly mammogram. The older a female is, the greater her risk of cancer.

## Function

Female breasts serve two purposes. They are a sexual part of the female adult body that produces pleasurable feelings when touched, and when females become pregnant, breasts produce milk for their babies. Some women enjoy breast feeding; others don't and they elect to feed their babies bottled formula. When a woman is pregnant her breasts become larger as they fill with breast milk. If the female doesn't breast-feed, the breast milk will dry up and the woman's breasts will return to their normal size. To breast-feed or not is a matter of personal choice.

The important point to remember is that most girls see their breasts as an important part of their anatomy. Girls worry about breast size, the same as guys worry about penis size. It's rude and mean to tease a girl about her breasts, just as you don't care to be teased about penis size or erections.

Most people enjoy being complimented on their appearance, but compliments should always be given in good taste. A comment like, "Whoa, what knockers," is *never* appropriate. A more appropriate compliment would be, "Great dress!" Though we are physically attracted to each other, it's always better manners to compliment someone's clothing rather than a specific body part. The exception to this is a couple in an intimate, long-term relationship talking privately to each other.

One other note about breasts . . . because of sex in advertising today, far too much emphasis has been placed on "large breasts." The truth is that breasts are nice whatever the size. If you won't date a girl because of her breast size, you don't deserve to date her, because you're concerned with her anatomy rather than the person. Likewise, girls shouldn't date guys as sex objects.

## Bras

Girls wear bras for the same reasons guys wear jock straps. Bras support breasts much like a jock strap gives a guy's penis and scrotum support. Some girls worry that their breasts will sag if they don't wear a bra, but girls shouldn't have to worry about sagging unless they have large breasts and they don't wear a bra for many years. Having children will cause women to lose some firmness in their breasts.

Bras are available in different sizes and styles, including extra-support "sports bras" for girls who participate in sports. Bra size is determined by cup size represented by a letter and the number of inches around the chest. For example, a 34B bra size means the cup size is B and the chest size is thirty-four inches. Cup sizes run from A through E and include AAA sizes for small breasts and EE sizes for large breasts. Chest sizes range from twenty-eight to forty-four inches.

## Body Hair

Hair growth may begin as early as age eight or as late as age sixteen. Like guys, females grow hair under their arms, on

### Five Stages of Pubic Hair Growth

Stage 1
Mons is hairless or there are a few light-colored soft hairs similar to arm hair.

State 2
A few darker-colored, somewhat curly hairs appear on the mons.

State 3
More hair appears and it is thicker, curlier and darker.

Stage 4
Hair spreads out in a triangular shape, still dark, thick, and curly.

State 5
Adult stage. Pubic hair covers a wider area than stage four and is thick and very curly. For some, pubic hair grows onto the thighs and/or toward the bellybutton (navel).

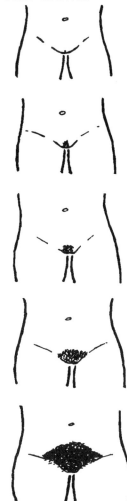

their legs, and pubic hair on their mons (the mound of skin between their legs). There are five stages of pubic hair growth for girls. As you can see these stages are similar to the stages of pubic hair growth in males.

Generally, in the United States, male body hair is considered attractive while female body hair is not considered attractive. Most women in America routinely remove underarm and leg hair (though generally not pubic hair, except for bikini lines). However, there are some women in America who keep their body hair. It's a matter of personal choice. In many countries women never shave and they are considered very sexy. If a female does remove underarm and leg hair, she usually does it in one of three ways.

Shaving is the least expensive way for women to remove body hair, but women also use chemical creams, waxing and electrolysis. Women use disposable, reusable, or electric razors and shaving is similar for both women and men.

## Female Outer Genital Area

A female's vulva (exterior genitals) includes the mons, clitoris, major and minor labia, and vaginal opening. The urinary and

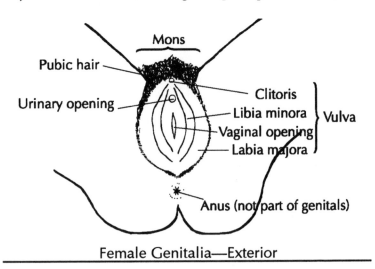

Female Genitalia—Exterior

intestinal outer organs included the urinary opening and anus, which we'll talk about later. A females reproductive system has many different parts and functions so you need to read this section carefully.

## Mons

Mons are the same in both boys and girls; it's the pad of fat tissue covering the pubic bone on which pubic hair grows.

## Labia

For the female, the mons actually continues downward where it divides into two separate soft folds of skin called the labia, which is Latin for lips. The labia are a covering for the clitoris and vaginal and urinary openings. There are two labia—labia majora (outside major lips) and labia minora (inside minor lips).

## Clitoris

The clitoris is a small but highly touch-sensitive organ of nerves and tissue located where the mons and labia meet. The clitoris is actually made up of the clitoral hood, shaft and glans. Whereas males experience orgasm by stimulation of the penis, females experience orgasm by stimulation of the clitoris. The clitoris is the female's most sensitive area of sexual pleasure.

The only part of the clitoris that can easily be seen is the clitoral glans which looks and feels like a small button or bump. Female orgasm is most often achieved through stimulation of the clitoris by partner massage, masturbation, oral contact, or intercourse.

## Urinary and Intestinal Systems

Female and male intestinal systems, ending with the rectum and anus, are identical, but the female urinary system is different. While males urinate and ejaculate from the penis, the urinary and vaginal openings in females are distinctly separate body parts. The urethra expels urine through the urinary opening. The vaginal opening is separate and has only reproductive functions.

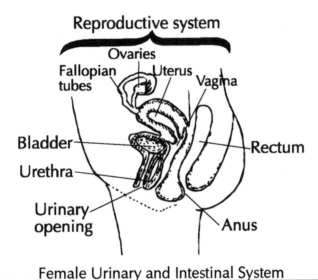

Female Urinary and Intestinal System

## Reproductive System

The female interior reproductive system is nature's way of enabling humans to develop new life. The system consists of the ovaries, fallopian tubes, uterus, cervix, and vagina.

When a girl's body begins changing into an adult body, usually between ages nine and sixteen, she begins ovulation—the process where her ova (eggs) mature. Just as you begin to produce sperm, a girl's reproductive system begins to mature and release her stored ova. Whereas males begin making sperm at the onset of puberty, females are born with their ova—thousands of tiny egg cells, of which only a few hundred will mature in a lifetime.

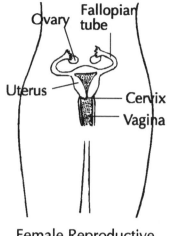

Female Reproductive System—Internal

### Ovaries

The ovaries are the sex organs where the woman's part of the reproductive process begins. When fully-grown, a woman's ovaries will be about the size of her thumb nail.

For most females ovulation is a monthly cycle during which the body matures an ovum which can be fertilized by male sperm to achieve conception and pregnancy. Once a month an ovum matures and bursts from one of the ovaries, where it is swept up by the tiny hairs on the end of the fallopian tube.

In a regular cycle, the ovaries take turns maturing an ovum each month. If one ovary is damaged or for a medical reason has to be removed, the other ovary takes over reproductive function in much the same way that a male testicle takes over sperm production if the other testicle is damaged.

If the ovum (egg cell) is not fertilized by male sperm,

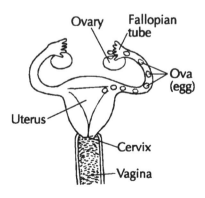

Route of the Egg

once a month the ovum and the endometrium (a blood-rich bed of tissue to nurture fertilized ovum) in the female's uterus dissolves and she menstruates (gets her monthly period).

If the ovum is fertilized by sperm, the fertilized ovum is called a zygote, and it travels down a fallopian tube to the uterus.

Twins occur when two ova ripen at the same time and are fertilized by two sperm (fraternal, non-identical twins-boy/ girl, girl/girl or boy/boy); or when a single zygote (ovum/ sperm union) splits into two zygotes (identical twins—boy/ boy or girl/girl).

## Fallopian tubes

The Fallopian tubes, no bigger than two strings of spaghetti, are the passageways from the ovaries to the uterus. When an ovum bursts from an ovary it takes four days for it to travel down a fallopian tube to reach the uterus. Usually for a pregnancy to occur, the ovum is fertilized by a sperm while in the fallopian tube.

## Uterus

The uterus (womb) is the organ where a fetus develops and the organ from which the menstrual flow (period) starts.

Each month, in a regular menstrual cycle, the uterus builds up endometrium . If the ovum reaching the uterus is not fertilized, the ovum and endometrium are expelled through the vagina and a female has her period.

If the ovum is fertilized by a sperm, the zygote (sperm-ovum union) attaches itself to the uterus, where if conditions are right, and it is allowed to develop, it will grow into a baby.

Fourteen days after conception (sperm fertilizing the ovum), the zygote is termed an embryo. At eight weeks human features become apparent and the embryo is called a fetus. Normally, an adult female's uterus is only about the size of a woman's fist. During pregnancy the uterus expands up to ten times its normal size to house and protect a seven or nine pound baby. Some pregnancies require that the uterus house twins (two babies) and more rarely three or more babies. After childbirth, the uterus contracts back to nearly its original size.

## Cervix

The cervix, at the lower part of the uterus, protrudes into the vagina. The cervix opening, called the "os," is about the size of the head of a pin and it is the gateway through which sperm swim into the uterus. During childbirth, this same opening stretches wide enough to allow a baby to pass through the cervix and into the birth canal (vagina). When a woman is pregnant, a small mucus plug forms in the opening of the cervix to protect the pregnancy from outside infections.

## Vagina

The vagina is an amazing passageway of strong, elastic muscles that leads to the uterus from outside of the body. An adult female's vagina is about three to five inches long and its muscular sides are collapsed together. But the vagina is very tough and elastic. It can expand to accommodate the male penis during intercourse, then expand large enough to allow a baby to pass through during childbirth; yet, when the muscles are collapsed together it is small enough to hold a tampon in place to soak up menstrual flow.

The vagina is normally clean and infection free, although it can become infected by a sexually-transmitted disease or irritated by an allergic reaction to a contraceptive cream or jelly. Women must be very careful not to contract sexually transmitted diseases, because STDs can travel up the vagina and into the uterus and fallopian tubes and damage them. This damage may cause a woman to become sterile (unable to have children).

Cleaning of the vagina is easy because it cleans itself. In earlier times, some doctors advised women to clean their vaginas by douching—flushing their vaginas with water, water-vinegar, or commercial solutions. That's why companies sell douches. Today, doctors know that a woman's vagina is self-cleaning. Unless douching is prescribed by a doctor for medical reason, douching may actually promote infections and rob the vagina of its self-cleaning ability.

### Hymen

The hymen (slang: cherry or maidenhead) is a thin piece of skin that usually covers part or all of a female's vaginal opening. Some women are born without hymens. The hymen can be a solid covering with one big hole in it, many small holes, or it may be a thin fringe of skin around the outside of the

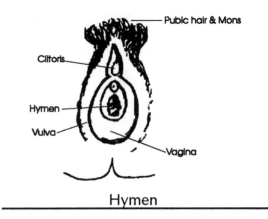

Hymen

opening. The illustration below shows only one type of hymen. The hymen usually stays intact until a woman's first sexual intercourse or tampon use, but sometimes strenuous exercise can break the hymen.

In earlier times, society demanded that a woman remain a virgin (person who hasn't had intercourse) until her wedding night—although, quite unfairly, those same rules didn't apply to men. Supposedly, a man could tell that his bride was a virgin on her wedding night if there was blood on the bed sheets, from his penis having broken the hymen.

Today we know that not all females have hymens, and hymens can be stretched or broken by tampons or vigorous exercise without intercourse having taken place. And besides that, it's no ones business but the bride and groom if they are or aren't virgins when they marry.

When a girl's hymen is first stretched or torn by tampons, exercise or intercourse it may hurt (and bleed) a little, a lot, or not at all. After the first complete tearing or stretching, any discomfort should disappear. If the hymen bleeds excessively or a girl has extreme pain she should see a doctor.

## Menstruation—A Girl's Monthly Period

It's important for you to know about the female menstrual cycle for two reasons:

1) you need to know how to prevent unwanted pregnancy during intercourse, because a woman can become pregnant anytime during her menstrual cycle—even when she's having her period;

2) when you begin dating, and if you eventually marry, knowing about a woman's hormonal changes will help you cope with those times during the month when your wife may be more emotional or moody than usual.

Girls normally start ovulation between eleven and seventeen years of age, and their periods come in monthly cycles or menstrual cycles. A cycle is the time from the first day of bleeding of one period to the first day of bleeding of the next period. The average menstrual cycle is about twenty-eight days, but cycles can range from twenty-one to thirty-five days.

Just as the length of the cycle varies, so does the length and amount of bleeding. From puberty to menopause having a period is a normal female body function. The blood flow ranges from one to three tablespoons per period. The average period lasts five days, though periods can range from two to seven days.

Periods aren't fun for girls, but they don't have to be a big hassle either. If a girl uses tampons or sanitary napkins correctly, no one has to know she's having her period.

To absorb the blood during their periods, girls use tampons, sanitary pads or napkins, or special menstrual sponges. These pads, tampons, and special sponges are small and absorbent so girls can continue their regular activities. Tampons and pads are made of soft absorbent cotton and both work well soaking up menstrual flow. Some women prefer pads, others prefer tampons. Because a girl never knows exactly when her

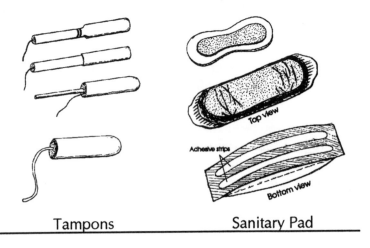

Tampons                    Sanitary Pad

period will come, pads and tampons are wrapped in plastic wrappers or discreet carrying pouches that a girl can tuck into her purse or book bag.

## A girl getting her first period

For a girl, getting that first period can be as awkward as when you have your first wet dream or spontaneous erection. That's why it's important that boys and girls respect each other's privacy and awkward moments, and don't tease each other about periods, erections, or other puberty experiences.

## Missed periods

When a girl first starts her periods, it's quite normal for them to be irregular. She may have them two weeks apart or miss several months between periods. Within a year her ovaries should settle into a regular monthly cycle, or she may be a woman who only has periods once every three to six months—and that will be normal for her.

Missed periods are cause for concern if a couple has had intercourse, they think their birth control method failed, and if the girl has symptoms of a pregnancy. However, worry, stress, and strenuous physical activity can also delay periods. The rule is: if a female is having intercourse and her period is supposed to come but she's fourteen days or more late, she should have a pregnancy test.

## How girls deal with their periods

Monthly periods don't have to interrupt a girl's social life. Most girls can do everything they normally do during their periods, including sports, school activities, swimming— anything that doesn't cause them discomfort.

During their periods, girls may experience mild cramps, stomach aches, breast tenderness, feel bloated, or feel somewhat grumpy. But unless a girl suffers from severe cramps or severe PMS (pre-menstrual syndrome) having her period generally won't slow her down.

## Menstruation affects female emotions

One important point that guys need to know about girls, is that the female reproductive system is controlled by a complicated set of hormones. Hormones affect emotional feelings in both men and women, but the female hormonal system is more complicated than the male system. Because of this, once a girl begins menstruation, she may be moody or more emotional at different times of the month—depending on where she is in her ovulation cycle.

Hormonal change isn't fun but it's something that all females live with. We appreciate males who are understanding and considerate when our hormones are exploding beyond our control. When your girlfriend is moody, the best thing to do is to ignore it and don't take it personally.

## Menopause

Women can become pregnant until they stop ovulating, normally between forty-five and fifty-five years of age. This aging change is called menopause; the brain quits sending signals to the ovaries to mature ovum. Menopause can happen quickly, over a period of months, or take years. But menopause does not mean a woman's sex life is over. If she or her partner don't develop health problems, men and women can enjoy intercourse their entire lives.

*Mom,*

*Do girls like having periods and having to deal with pregnancy? It sounds like periods are a big hassle.*

You're right, Michael. Periods aren't fun. I've never met a female who liked having periods. But that's the way the procreation process is set up. We women handle periods, pregnancy, and the pain of childbirth because after delivery the someone we felt kicking us in the ribs is our very own brand new baby son or daughter. Being able to give birth to you and have you as my son is one of the reasons I'm glad I'm female.

Even though men don't get pregnant, supporting their wives through pregnancies and seeing their children born is an emotional experience. And being a dad to your child will be one of the most rewarding feelings in the world. If at all possible, every kid needs both an available dad and mom—male and female role models, teachers and nurturers.

Now you know about girls' bodies, ovulation, periods, conception, and pregnancy.

My next few letters are on dating. Why do girls and guys go together? Why do guys like girls. Why do girls like guys?

Take Care,
Mom

_____

_____

_____

_____

_____

_____

_____

_____

# LETTER 11

## DATING, THE BASICS

Dear Michael,

Why do people date? Why do guys like girls? Why do girls like guys? It's human nature.

Male and female being together is as old as the world. You begin dating because there is something that attracts you to a person. The girl you like may have beautiful eyes, a great smile, or a great body. You may be attracted to her because she's funny, cool, serious, or sexy.

Sometimes you can't even describe why you like someone; it's just how you feel. Why did I like your father? Why did he like me?

Teens told me that once they are attracted to each other, they date for many reasons:

- They date to get to know each other better.
- They date for fun.
- They date for romance.
- They date to feel grown-up.

- They date to find out what personality traits they like and dislike in people.

Later on, people date to find a committed partner, for marriage, and to raise children together.

Unfortunately, people also date for the wrong reasons such as dating for status or dating for sex. You date someone because she's popular in school or she's especially good-looking, but you don't really care about her. Maybe she's dating you for the same reason. Other teens date to boost their self-esteem or in the hope of finding the love and attention they aren't getting from home.

The most important reasons to date are that dating gives you experience dealing with relationships and teaches what makes a relationship work. You date to get to know a person better and find out if you and she are compatible—and, dating is usually fun.

## Three Stages of Teen Dating

### Stage 1: Junior high/middle school

Normally, guys and girls start liking each other and going together in junior high or middle school. But because you can't drive yet, your time together is limited to school and after school activities.

Junior high "going together" is usually short-term dating because guys and girls aren't yet comfortable with dating. A girl may want to go together one week but the next week change her mind and break up. You may do the same thing. Opinions from friends also play a part in who you date and don't date. These opinions often change weekly, further shortening middle school relationships.

### Stage 2: Freshman/sophomore years

During freshman and sophomore years of high school, girls and guys continue to be interested in dating. High school relationships generally last longer than junior high dating, but long-term commitments of one or more years aren't yet the norm. You are still learning about going together and your likes and dislikes. During your teens you may be attracted to girls younger, older, or the same age as you.

For guys, there can be a couple of serious dating problems: girls who keep hounding guys and won't leave them alone and girls who trick guys into a teen pregnancy.

A worry every parent has is that their son will have sex, he won't use birth control, and he'll get a girl pregnant. State law requires child support. If, as a teen, you get a girl pregnant and she keeps the baby, you will pay child support until your child is eighteen, regardless of whether you choose to participate in raising the child. Having a child when you are married is great, but finding out at sixteen that you are a teen dad is not cool.

Most of your relationships will be good ones. But in every relationship make sure the girl is dating you for you. The majority of girls are honest and sincere, but some girls (like some guys) don't have great home lives. Girls who aren't getting parental love from home often try to substitute sex for love. They may trick a guy into getting them pregnant because they think a baby will bring them love.

Two of the worst sexual consequences that can happen to you in high school are a teen pregnancy and AIDS. Always be on your guard. I don't care how good looking a girl is or how sexually-aroused (slang: horny, turned-on) you are—respect yourself. Don't let yourself get in a bad relationship or have sex without birth control—not even one time. Relationships are about caring, trust, respect, and honesty. Anything less and you will get hurt.

Stage 3: Junior/senior years

By your junior and senior years of high school:

- you may be going with someone, or
- you've had it with girls and you're hanging around with your friends waiting for life after high school, or you have a group of guy and girl friends you do things with.

Probably, by your senior year you will have formed some opinions of what does and doesn't make a good date and a good relationship.

How do you know if a girl is worth dating or not? One way is the dolphin versus shark test. Dolphins are intelligent, gentle, and fun to be with. Sharks are sly, aggressive, selfish scavengers, who take whatever they can get. The same is true in dating. Some people are dolphins, others are sharks.

When you start liking a girl or she starts liking you, take a good look at her. See if she matches the shark list or the dolphin list. Go for the dolphins. Stay away from the sharks. Sharks are only out for themselves. They get what they want from a guy and dump him.

| SHARKS | DOLPHINS |
|---|---|
| 1. Big Egos | 1. Intelligent |
| 2. Aggressive | 2. Kind |
| 3. Deceiving | 3. People Oriented |
| 4. Sleek/polished | 4. Good-looking |
| 5. Attack People | 5. Helpers |
| 6. Scavengers | 6. Joiners |
| 7. Selfish | 7. Loving, Faithful |
| 8. Dresses In Dolphin's Clothes | 8. Always Themselves |

*Mom, at what age can I date?*

Michael, each family has different guidelines for dating. Many families still adhere to fifteen or sixteen as a mature age to date, but they allow their sons and daughters in middle school to meet friends at the movies, the mall, or school activities.

Since you asked about dating, we'll have to sit down and talk about it. We would also like to meet the girls you date. We're not being nosey; we're genuinely interested in meeting the girls you like.

Once you get your driver's license you can car date. But we will have to decide on a reasonable time for you to come home from your dates. If you date an older girl who drives before you get your license, there will also be a home time for those dates.

I know home time, (often called a curfew) can seem like parents are being totally unfair. But home time isn't a plot to keep you from having fun. Home time is a safeguard.

Michael, I love you more than anything else in the world, even those times I forget to tell you. A parent's greatest fear when their teens begin car dating or riding in a car with friends is that they'll be involved in a car accident or other serious trouble and be hurt or killed.

Teens under age twenty rate the highest number of accidental car deaths in any age group. A teen dies in a car accident every eleven minutes. More than fifty percent of all traffic deaths involve a drunk driver or a driver on drugs.

Home time is a safeguard to help protect you against drunk drivers and decrease the chance that you or a friend will fall asleep at the wheel and end up in a ditch. I loved going out with my friends when I was a teen. Looking back now, I'm glad my parents loved me enough to give me a home time, so I didn't end up hurt or dead.

But let's move on to more cheerful subjects. My next letter to you is a long one and it's full of all sorts of dating and relationship information. You can be sure it will be good reading.

I love you,

Mom

_____

_____

_____

_____

_____

_____

_____

_____

# Letter 12

# Dating, Relationships, and Friends

Dear Michael,

When a guy and a girl start dating or going together, they've entered into a relationship. From the time you start dating and you are involved with a girl you are in a relationship.

Relationship is defined in Webster's Dictionary as: the state of being "mutually" interested or involved with one another. Mutually means both the guy and girl equally like and care for each other, and it's one of the qualities of a good relationship. However, many people have never been taught the qualities of a good relationship. Others grapple with self-esteem issues.

Some people date because that's how they maintain self-esteem. They only know how to feel good about themselves through other people. Using dating for self-love is destructive. It's a false high that destroys self-worth.

At times in your life you will wrestle with your self-esteem. Everyone does. When something is troubling you, you don't feel good. But talking it out with someone often helps. I'm always available and will listen, and you can talk to close friends. If you can't work out your dilemma with my or a friend's help, seek professional help from a school counselor or psychologist.

The things that make you a good person are your smile, sense of humor, honor, loyalty to friends, and caring attitude. Each of us is a great human being; we just don't realize it sometimes.

A relationship will not solve life's problems, but it should be a positive addition to your life. Here is a checklist of qualities a good relationship should have. Use it to evaluate whether a relationship is good.

* You both feel good about dating each other. Neither of you is embarrassed to have people know that you are dating.

* You can talk to each other and share private thoughts.

* You have similar values and beliefs.

* You respect each other. You focus on each other's good points rather than weaknesses.

* You both care for and equally support each other.

* You have interests together and apart from each other. You like being together, but you don't have to be with each other every minute of the day.

* You may argue and disagree, but you can both laugh at your disagreements afterward.

* Your relationship is not verbally or physically abusive. Neither of you beat, hit, or yell at each other.

* You both realize that a relationship means compromise, each partner caring for the other partner's welfare.

For a relationship to have a chance, positive qualities must be evident within the first few meetings and long-term relationships take time to develop—weeks, months, years.

The majority of middle school and high school dating is short-term. You are learning about relationships and what personality types you are compatible with. The following are different situations most everyone will experience at one time or another. I hope reading about them will help you in similar situations.

## You Like a Girl But She Isn't Interested In You

This is an age-old problem. You like a girl, but she isn't interested in you. When you like someone but find out she's not interested, you may have feelings of disappointment or frustration. You may put yourself down, thinking you are not interesting or good-looking.

Your Dad said when he was in high school, he liked a number of girls who wouldn't give him the time of day—brains, cheerleaders, rockers. He'd ask a girl out and she'd look at him like he was from another planet. On the other hand, he said there were girls who chased him and he wasn't interested in them.

When I was in high school, there were a number of guys I wanted to date, but they weren't interested in me. I'd get excited about a guy, and he didn't even know I existed. Have you had experiences like this with girls?

If a girl isn't interested in you it means the two of you aren't meant to be together at that time. There is someone else for you. Sometimes it's impossible to believe there could be anyone else. But there is and she's usually waiting around the next corner.

## Getting a Girl to Like You

You can't. You simply can't. People are attracted to each other or they aren't. You can get a girl to notice you by spending time where she spends time or working on a project together, but you can't make another person like you. You only cause yourself disappointment and pain trying to make happen that which isn't meant to be.

## Telling a Girl You Are Not Interested In Her

Michael, telling someone "I like you as a person, but I'm not attracted to you as someone to date" can be very difficult. It's a conversation you may have many times in your life. The best way to tell someone is straight out in a firm, honest way without making excuses and without putting them down. For example:

"Chelsie, you're good-looking and fun, but I'm not attracted to you as someone to date. I'd rather be truthful with you than make excuses. I'm sorry but our going out won't work."

When the time comes to tell a girl you aren't attracted to her, how do you think you'll say it?

## Liking Two Girls at the Same Time

What do you do if you are attracted to two girls at once? This happens to a lot of people and it may happen at different times throughout your life. In most schools, it's difficult if not impossible to date both girls at once. There is a sort of unwritten rule that you only date one person at a time.

It's hard when you like two girls at once. Look at your potential relationship with each girl. Do both girls seem genuine, trustworthy, caring, and honest? Does one seem a better choice than the other? Are you attracted to one slightly more than the other? What do you do? You have to choose. Date one girl and see how it works out. If you break up and the other girl still wants to go out, date her and see how that works. Eventually relationship situations always work themselves out.

## Talking to Your Date

Communicating (listening and sharing) is the essence of relationships. Communicating is sharing yourself with another *person. It can be the toughest job in the world. In dating (and marriage) it's always easier to kiss someone than to tell them what that kiss means. Is that kiss friendship, like, love, or lust?*

Communicating is tough because it's sharing your personality and inner feelings with someone. That's scary because that person may not accept you. But you have to take the risk. If you don't communicate, you don't have intimacy and you don't have a relationship—whether it's friendship or a dating relationship. The following suggestions may help.

• Take it slow. Ask the person out for a date. Talk about school, movies, music, sports, family, dreams, or goals. Listen to your date when she is talking. If you are shy and find it hard to talk, write down a list of things you could talk about. Practice talking in a mirror at home before you go out on the date. It may seem awkward practicing in front of a mirror, but it should help you feel more at ease—especially if she's a girl you really like. List some things you could talk about with her.

• If you realize on the first date that you aren't right for each other, you can go your separate ways. You have each learned something about yourselves. No harm done.

• If you both like the first date, be honest with each other about your feelings and make plans to go out again.

• Remember. You have to take a risk to develop any dating relationship or friendship.

## Asking a Girl Out or Telling a Girl You Like Her

The best way to ask someone out is to call her or talk to her at school. If you are shy, ask a trusted friend to let the girl know you like her.

## When a Girl Turns You Down for a Date

This is called rejection and it may happen many times in your life. Not everyone you are attracted to is going to be attracted to you. It's the same for a girl who likes you, but you aren't attracted to her.

You really wanted to go out with this girl. She turned you down. You're hurt or embarrassed. You want to avoid her. That's okay. After a turn down everyone needs time to muster their self-esteem again. Girls feel the same way when they ask you out and you're not interested.

The best thought I have about asking a girl out is this: if you like her, take the chance. If she turns you down, it doesn't mean you're not good-looking. It's no reason to give up dating. Maybe in a year or so, she will go out with you. Meanwhile, go on with life. Keep your eyes open to meeting the next someone special.

During your teens it's likely that you will turn girls down for dates, and you will also be turned down possibly many times. Does this mean you should withdraw from the human race, lock yourself in your room, and forget life? Absolutely not. It means you try again. Risk and fail. Risk and win.

## Paying for the Date

I'm giving you my personal thoughts on this, Michael. Who pays depends on the circumstances of the date, individual finances, and informal dating rules at your school. You will have to decide what is best in each relationship.

For teens with a limited income or allowance, dating can be expensive. Many teens have groups of friends that go out together and each person pays her or his own way.

I think on a first date (perhaps the first few dates) the person who does the asking out should pay for the date.

If you decide to keep dating, talk to each other about how to handling dating expenses. Be honest with the girl. If you are short on money, tell her you want to keep dating, but you don't have a lot of money. Tell her you'll be able to go to movies or participate in other activities that cost money occasionally but not every week.

Today, girls who have a part time job or allowance will often offer to help with the expenses. You buy the movie tickets, she buys the drinks and popcorn.

Be sure that both of you are agreeable on who pays what share.

+ Who works? You, she, both, neither?

+ Who has more "play" money?

+ Are either of you old-fashioned and feel the male should always pay? Do you need to compromise?

+ What method feels comfortable to you and your date?

+ When talking about money: Offer only what you can afford. It's easy to feel generous and over commit yourself. If you do spend too much one week, admit it to your partner. Tell her you will have to do something inexpensive next weekend, like renting a video and watching it at home.

+ If money problems arise, don't be afraid to talk to each other. Money misunderstandings can quickly ruin a relationship.

+ Be flexible to one another's job changes or other situations which affect available income.

+ Every date does not have to be an expensive affair. You can rent videos. In the summer there is the beach, the zoo, or the park.

- You never "owe" a date sex, or anything else when they pay for the date. A date is a date, not a payment for sexual activity. Likewise, you are not to expect sex or other favors for spending money on a person. Dating is about mutual respect for each other, whoever pays.

## When Guys and Girls Lead Each Other On

Males and females should always respect each other. Both sexes can feel the pain of a deception or rejection. It's not right for guys or girls to use each other. But sometime, when you want something, it's easy to forget your values just this one time.

In high school I wanted to go to a concert. I knew a guy who liked me, and I knew he'd take me. I didn't like him but I wanted to see the concert. Your grandma told me that I wasn't being fair to him, but I left my conscience at home and went to the concert. He paid for everything and of course assumed that I went with him because I liked him.

The next week he called me for another date and I had to tell him I didn't want to date him. After that, he wouldn't look at me in the halls. I knew he was hurt, I felt like dirt. I didn't like people using me, but I had used him.

What could I have done differently? I could have paid my own way and gone to the concert with a girlfriend. I could have made it clear I only liked him as a friend and paid for half of everything. In dating you learn a lot about life. I learned a good lesson.

A situation like this could happen to you. Suppose you ask a girl to a dance only because you want to go and you need a date. She thinks you really like her. Or a girl goes with you only because she needs a date to the dance and then drops you afterward.

Sexually, it's also easy to lead someone on. When you are sexually aroused (turned-on, horny) it's easy to forget your self-respect and respect for others.

Your sexuality is an extremely powerful force. A poll taken at one high school revealed that 90 percent of the guys said that when they were sexually excited, they would tell a girl anything to make out or have sex with her. Though many said they didn't like themselves for being dishonest, they gave in to their physical wants. This is wrong—and in the case of rape or sexual abuse it's a crime.

When you lead another person on for sexual activity or any other personal gain, you don't respect yourself—and neither do others respect you. Likewise, girls should not lead guys on. Some do and it's wrong. Anytime you find yourself in either situation, stop. Leave the situation. Walk away. The bottom line is: don't lead other people on, and don't fall for someone who is leading you on.

## Girlfriends Are Not Problem Fixers

Michael, everyone has personal or family problems during their lives. It's easy to want someone—a friend or girlfriend—to fix the problem, take us away from it, and take care of us. But a girlfriend isn't a mother or a big sister who will help you solve problems. That type of relationship isn't healthy. Good relationships are not based on dependence.

## Unhealthy or Abusive Relationships

No human being deserves to be abused. If you get into a relationship with a girl who is mean to you, hits you, calls you names, or is too daring for you, get out of the relationship. If a girl is abusive, she isn't good for you.

Likewise, guys do not have the right to abuse their girlfriends. Everyone has personal problems in his/her life, but no one has the right to inflict their problems on another person.

Among teens today, there is an increase in the number of guys physically abusing their girlfriends. This is wrong. It seems if a guy gets mad, or his girlfriend wants to break up and he doesn't, or he gets jealous, he beats on the girl. Teens raised in abusive homes may think abuse is normal behavior. The truth is abuse is a crime, punishable by law.

Any time a teen couple finds themselves arguing and fighting most of the time they're together, they need to take a good look at the relationship. Discuss what's causing the problem. Perhaps one person wants to break up but is afraid and masks the unhappiness in fighting and nit-picking. Sometimes one of the partners may be jealous (with or without good reason) and that's the reason for fighting.

Whatever the problem, a relationship isn't a fighting match. A relationship is caring for one another and enjoying time spent with one another.

If you get into a bad relationship, *get out immediately and don't go back*. If you have problems controlling your anger in relationships, go to a school counselor or county health clinic and get help.

In school you go together and break up and go together and break up. In junior high you may not go with a girl more than two or three weeks. That's not enough time to even start a relationship. In junior high and high school all the going together and breaking up can become frustrating and make your life complicated. That's normal.

If you want to increase your chances of having good relationships take to heart these eight points.

* Each of us counts as a human being. Each of us wants to have good friendships and relationships, and each of us has the potential for good friendships and relationships.

* There is no life rule that says you must have a girlfriend all the time. That's like saying all guys must wear tattoos.

Maybe you are a person who has more fun with a group of friends. What you do is right for you.

+ Date only if you really like the girl. Dating to gain acceptance or status at school or to fill a void of family love or self-esteem isn't healthy for you, and it's not fair to the girl.

+ If you like someone but they don't like you, it doesn't mean you're unattractive or uninteresting. It means that the two of you aren't meant to be together right now. There is someone else for you.

+ You cannot make someone like you or love you. Yes, you can hang around that person more and make sure you're noticed, but, in the end, a person will either be attracted to you or not be attracted to you.

+ If you get hurt by a relationship or friendship, prolonging your hurt only puts your life on hold. You need to mourn, so go ahead and let out your anger or tears in a safe manner that won't hurt you or others. Then pick yourself up and get on with your life. There will be other relationships for you.

+ Relationships require communication. Friendships, dating, and marriage work only when both people in the relationship communicate with each other.

+ The best relationships often happen when a person isn't looking for someone. Your Aunt Celia appeared when your Uncle Derrick had had it with girls.

Except for about one percent of the teen population, teen relationships aren't forever. Your teens and early twenties are for learning about relationships so it's normal to date several different people and make mistakes.

## Guy/Girl Friendships

Some guys have best friends who are girls. This can be someone you've grown up with whom you've been friends with for many years, or it may be someone you met at school. She may be your age, younger, or older. You can talk to each other about anything including each other's dating dilemmas. Best friends are great. Not every guy has a girl for a best friend, but if you do that's something special.

The only problem you may need to watch for is that sometimes dates become jealous of best friends. The best approach to jealousy is for you and your friend to respect the concerns of the date while assuring her that the relationship is simply a friendship. Hopefully, the date will be able to accept the friendship.

## When Best Friends Date

What if one of you suddenly develops a romantic interest in the other? Michael, this is a tough situation and it happens quite often.

Most of the people I've talked to said their experience of dating a best friend in high school didn't turn out well. It wrecked the friendship for awhile.

On the other hand, I know of two best friends who started dating after high school. The couple married and their marriage is great. If you and your female best friend start dating and it doesn't work out, the friendship may be temporarily hurt. But if it is a strong friendship, down the road you should come back to being friends.

## When Best Friends Have Sex With Each Other

I'd say do not have sex with your best friend. This is how one teen summed it up:

My best friend asked me to have sex with her. I said okay (we both wanted to see what it was like). Afterward our friendship wasn't the same. I thought we could keep having sex as friends. She couldn't handle that. We started avoiding each other. I missed being her friend. It's been a whole year and we're just now starting to talk to each other again. I hope our friendship comes back to what it was before. I never want to have sex with a best friend again, it just messes things up.

The only exception to this is when occasionally two friends finish high school and realize they are attracted to each other. In their twenties they may make the decision to turn their friendship into a dating relationship.

## When Best Friends Grow Apart

Guy/girl friendships change just like other types of friendships. Your best friend in junior high may not be your best friend in high school. Change can hurt, but for every old friend who moves on, there are new friends to take her or his place.

Michael, I hope I've given you some reasonable standards you can use to judge the quality of your relationships. Let me know if you have any questions about this letter.

My next letter to you is titled Going Together and Breaking Up. I think you will find it good reading.

Here's to good relationships,

Mom

_____

_____

_____

_____

_____

# LETTER 13

# Going Together and Breaking Up

Dear Michael,

Going together is nice; breaking up feels lousy. Being liked by someone you like feels wonderful; liking someone who is not interested in you hurts. But all these interactions are part of having relationships.

If everyone took a course entitled *Relationships* in junior high, high school, and then again as adults, perhaps we'd all be better at relationships—dating relationships, friendships, and marriage. I hope the following information will be helpful to you.

## Going Together

Teens today say "going together" basically means the same as when I was a teen. Going together means dating only one person at a time. Once a couple has a few dates, it's thought of as going together until they break up.

Going together equals a relationship. Couples can have good or bad relationships. If both partners practice the principles of a good relationship (see Letter 10), going together can be great.

If one or both partners are still learning about relationships, going together can be frustrating and troublesome.

Teen dating provides you with valuable lessons in self-esteem, love, lust, jealousy, and possessiveness during one of the rockiest periods of your life. Some of these lessons will be painful. Have you ever needed to bounce back from a painful experience?

The following situations are not uncommon when you are in a going together relationship.

## You think your girlfriend is cheating on you

First, try to find out if the information is true. This can be tough because the information could be a rumor started by someone who wants you to break up.

If you have evidence that makes you suspect she is cheating on you, schedule some time alone with her. Calmly (not accusingly) tell her you saw or heard things that lead you to think she's going out on you. It's important to keep a cool, level head while you're talking to her. Ask her if the information is true. Is she tired of going together? Does she want to break up? Wait for her to answer.

If she doesn't want to break up, tell her you expect her to stop whatever she's been doing immediately. If she wants to break up, the best thing to do is break up right then. Breaking up is tough, especially if you really like a girl. But if she's cheating on you she's not worth your time.

## You break up with a girl, she starts dating someone else, and you want her back

First, be sure you are not falsely jealous. If you genuinely want her back, you may let her know it. However, it's not right to go in and break up a relationship. She may not want to get back with you. If she does, great. If she doesn't, that hurts. You may have to steer clear of her until the hurt goes away.

## You like a girl who is going with someone else

Wait until they break up. It's not right to break up a relationship.

## A friend's girlfriend and you start liking each other

This is another tough situation. One person in the triangle is going to be hurt.

* Tell her he is your friend.

* Tell her if she breaks up with him to date you, she'll have to wait until he gets over the break up before you and she start dating.

* Tell her you won't date her behind his back.

This may be hard for both of you. But stop and ask yourself how you would feel if someone were dating your girlfriend behind your back?

These are relationship situations for you to think about. Although I'm sure I missed some, the important thing to remember is that if you're faced with a situation you don't know how to handle, ask for help—from me, a friend, a school counselor.

Your job is to learn and become stronger, not to crash and burn. You can do it! Each of us possesses a tough inner strength. If you call on your inner strength you can bounce back from any relationship. You can triumph over any life challenge.

## Breaking up

A popular song when I was a teen was "Breaking Up is Hard to Do!" Breaking up was and always will be difficult because being in a relationship means dealing with another's feelings as well as your own. Breaking up always hurts one or both partners.

What if you think you want to break up? First, make sure you really want to do it. Ask yourself the following questions. Write your answers down on paper. These questions also apply to friendships.

+ What first attracted you to your girlfriend?

+ What things do you like and dislike about her and your relationship at the present time?

+ If there is a problem, have you talked about it as a couple and tried to solve it?

+ Is breaking up something you want to do or are your friends or a situation influencing you?

+ Why do you want out of the relationship? Are you feeling smothered or wanting to date other people. Maybe there are sexual pressures or she's abusive.

Common reasons for breaking up are:

+ You don't want to be tied down. You want the chance to date around.

+ You're feeling smothered, partner too serious, need space.

+ You want to date someone else.

+ You aren't compatible. The relationship has stalled.

+ Your falling "out of love" (lust/infatuation is gone).

+ You are being pressured sexually or being physically or mentally abused.

If you decide to break up, how are you going to tell her? It depends on the relationship. If your girlfriend is calm and mature, breaking up in person may be best. If she has a temper, a phone call or letter may be better so she has a chance to cool off.

You'll probably want to create your own note, but here is an example of a written break up.

Dear Jenny,

I don't know how to write this except to tell you straight out that I want to break up. I'm sorry if this is a surprise.

I'm breaking up because . . . (include the reason you are breaking up in the kindest, gentlest way possible).

You are a good person. It's nothing you did or didn't do in the relationship. It's me. I just need out.

If this hurts, I'm sorry. It hurts me, too. Breaking up is hard. You will find someone else. There are other guys out there for you. It's best you find someone else. You may want to avoid me for awhile. That's OK. I understand. I don't mean to hurt you, but I know it hurts. Call me and let's talk. I'd like to say goodbye and know how you are doing.

### Your girlfriend wants to break up with you

This is a tough one. You may not want to break up. But it's better to confront her than hurt yourself by denying or avoiding the problem. Ask her in person, phone, or write her. This is a sample script. You write your own.

Dear Julie,

I've felt these last few weeks (days) that something is wrong between us. Is there a problem? Do you want to break up? If you do, tell me. I don't want to break up, but I need to know what's wrong.

Wait for her answer. If she doesn't want to break up, ask her what is bothering her. Is it a problem with the relationship or something personal? If it's a relationship problem, talk about how the two of you can solve it.

If she wants to break up, you'll want to know why. You deserve an answer because you are a part of the relationship, but she may not give you an answer or give you an honest answer. You may want to scream or cry.

Breaking up hurts. The process of getting over a relationship or friendship is similar to the process of resolving a death. There is a mourning process which can include all or some of these stages:

- Denial—She couldn't have dumped me like that!

- Anger—Why that no good..., I'll show her.

- Bargaining—If she'd come back, I'd. . . .

- Depression—I can't believe it's over. What went wrong?

- Acceptance—Okay, it's over. We weren't right for each other. There is someone else out there for me.

The hurt is real. It can feel like your whole world is falling apart. But your first breakup won't be the only one. The average male has hundreds of friendships and may have a number of relationships before finding his life partner. Life is too full to let one relationship get you down. You have to heal the hurt and get on with life.

When my eighth grade boyfriend broke up with me, I was angry and depressed for weeks. I was convinced no one loved me, and I would never find someone else. To make matters worse, my old boyfriend and his new girlfriend were around every corner I turned. Friends tried to comfort me, but I was convinced my life was ruined.

A month later a guy in band class started liking me. I found I liked him better than my first boyfriend. Now looking back on the situation, I see how I could have made things easier for myself. I shouldn't have wasted so much time being depressed. My old boyfriend wasn't the only guy on the earth. A new boyfriend did come into my life.

You could have the same situation happen to you. You and a girl break up. You feel like your life is over. A month later, you find out that someone else likes you. You start going out and find you like this girl more than your old girlfriend.

Sometimes in break up situations you need to avoid each other until the angry party has worked through the hurt. When I broke up with my freshman boyfriend, I wanted to be friends. But when I'd say, "Hi," he'd follow me around insisting we get back together. I knew he was hurt and not thinking rationally. Even though I didn't want to, I finally had to avoid him for awhile until he cooled off. Finally he started liking someone else. The interesting development was that by our senior year, though we were dating other people, we'd become close friends.

You may experience some of these same hurtful break ups in your lifetime. Readjustment time varies anywhere from a few days to several months to a year or more. Being obsessively depressed is dangerous; so is failing to grieve over your loss.

When you're feeling hurt, angry, or depressed, your body releases chemicals that add to those emotions. You can help yourself get over a break up faster by doing two things.

* Alternate your time between time with yourself and being around friends.

* Get regular daily exercise, such as walking, swimming, running, cycling, basketball, soccer, or other sport. Exercise releases chemicals in your brain which counteract the chemicals that are adding to your hurt.

I hope this letter is helpful to you in dealing with relationships. My next letter deals with the serious subject of sex in dating and should give you lots to think about.

Love you,

Mom

---

_____

_____

_____

_____

_____

_____

_____

_____

_____

# Letter 14

# Dating and Sex

Dear Michael,

How far should you go sexually when you date? This is a difficult question to answer. A couple will probably hold hands, kiss, and walk around arm in arm. The closer you are to a girl romantically the more your body says, "I want to be physically close to her."

The stronger the physical attraction the more your bodies will want to respond to each other. However, sexual activity encompasses many different levels. The decision concerning sexual involvement depends on:

- Your age
- How long you and your girlfriend have been dating
- How well you know each other
- Your beliefs about sexual activity
- Her beliefs about sexual activity
- Your maturity level
- Her maturity level

- Whether the relationship is a good friendship, crush, lust, or the beginning of a mutual like,

- Your reasons for wanting to respond physically to your girlfriend: you may want to show affection, caring, love, or she's good-looking and you're in lust (sexual attraction only)

There are five levels of sexual interaction.

(1) Kissing, hugging, holding hands

(2) Making out, prolonged kissing sessions

(3) Light petting, feeling body parts while clothed

(4) Heavy petting, exploring body parts under clothes or partially unclothed

(5) Intercourse, slang: having sex, making love, doing it, messing with, and oral-genital sex (slang: blow job, eating at the Y).

In Grandpa's high school days, social rules demanded that young people limit sexual activity in junior high to holding hands. Kissing, making out, and petting were for high school. Intercourse was for marriage.

By my teens, we were kissing in junior high. By high school graduation about one-third to one-half of the seniors had experienced intercourse. Today many more high school students will be sexually active. Parents believe that because of sex in movies, magazines, and on television, teens are experimenting sexually at much earlier ages.

Parents are concerned because:

- Teens aren't protecting themselves against STDs. STDs, AIDS, and teen pregnancy are serious threats to life, health, reproductivity, and sexuality.

- Many teens today aren't using birth control. Teen pregnancy rates have skyrocketed.

- Young teens aren't ready to handle the emotional feelings of intercourse. They don't understand the difference between sex and love.

Respecting your sexuality and that of others is important when you date. Intercourse is the most intimate way for two people to express their love for each other. Intercourse isn't something to pass around freely like a bag of junk food. Choose your relationships carefully. Don't date people who don't respect you and who aren't trustworthy and honest.

## Junior High/Middle School

Most parents feel that junior high/middle school couples should stick to kissing, holding hands, and making out.

Here are the reasons why:

- Middle school teens rarely use birth control or don't use it correctly.

- Having a multitude of sex partners increases your chances of contracting AIDS and other STDs and fathering a child. If you start having sex in middle school, there is a good chance you'll be a teen father before high school graduation. You may also contract AIDS for which there is currently no cure.

- Having sex in middle school is usually viewed as a game—have sex with someone and move on to a new partner. Sex-only dating can hurt you physically and emotionally.

## High School

In high school, the question of how far you go sexually depends on your moral convictions about sexual activity.

The heavier the making out, the greater the urge is to have intercourse. Petting (caressing body parts, partially clothed or unclothed) is actually the second of the four phases of intercourse. During heavy petting, the male's penis becomes erect and the female's vagina becomes moist. Your body's natural, physiological response is to have intercourse. Your body tries to override your mind. It's often difficult to stop yourself from going all the way—regardless of how moral or religious you are or how frightened you may be of AIDS, pregnancy, or STDs. If you are considering heavy petting, you need to know that it can lead to having sex.

Of the many persons you'll date, there will probably be only one or two with whom you could have a lasting intimate relationship. Most of us don't find that person or persons until our late teens or twenties.

When the time comes that you consider intercourse, be sure you are ready:

+ Are you having sex for reasons other than a loving and committed relationship? Some guys and girls have intercourse to be accepted at school. Some people drift into sexual activity without thinking and then become trapped with a pregnancy, STD, or AIDS.

+ Is this something you want to do, or is your girlfriend pressuring you to have sex? What are your beliefs about sexual activity?

+ Are you and your partner ready to handle the new feelings that can accompany intercourse: love, guilt, uncomfortableness, jealousy, possessiveness, embarrassment, and confusion?

+ What are the health risks? Is this the type of girl who's had sex with other guys before you? Condoms are good, but if the condom breaks you are at risk for making the girl pregnant and catching chlamydia, syphilis, gonorrhea, AIDS, or other STDs.

+ What if the girl becomes pregnant? Condoms alone are not 100% effective in preventing pregnancy. Is the girl on the pill, Norplant®, or using some other form of effective contraceptive? Without birth control, she can get pregnant anytime during her monthly cycle.

Three million sperm are released into the vagina on each ejaculation and it only takes one to make a girl pregnant. If she is on the pill, does she take it the same time daily, or does she skip days? Girls on the pill frequently get pregnant anyway because they don't take the pill correctly. For teens, a condom and the pill is better pregnancy prevention than the pill alone.

+ Is this someone with whom you have a long-term relationship or is this just one of many girls you'll date before marrying or settling down with one partner?

+ The greater the number of sexual partners you have, the greater your risk is for AIDS.

Can you show love without having sex?

Teens told me they have definite beliefs about sexual involvement. Some teens have religious beliefs about intercourse. They believe God intended intercourse for marriage only. Until they marry, they limit their sexual activity to kissing, hugging, holding hands, and making out.

Other teens have moral feelings about intercourse. They want heavy petting and intercourse to be with someone special, someone with whom they have a solid relationship. They know that person may not come along until sometime after high school, and they are willing to wait for the right relationship.

What do you think about these beliefs?

There are also teens who think casual intercourse is fine whenever and with whomever, it's a game. Some protect themselves and their partners from pregnancy, AIDS, and STDs, others don't. How do you feel about casual sex?

Sadly, a few teens never use contraceptive or STD protection. These guys and girls don't care if they spread STDs or AIDS or create a pregnancy. How do you feel about how these teens treat themselves and others?

Other teens have good morals, but they are in such need of parental-love or self-love that they get into sex in hopes of satisfying their love need. Unfortunately, sex alone isn't love. What do you think might help these teens?

Your sexuality is an extremely powerful force, Michael. A touch as simple as a kiss can be arousing. But sexual involvement is intimate, mature involvement. Having sex is similar to driving, voting, and drinking. You need a certain level of maturity to handle the responsibility.

If you and your girlfriend can't talk about sexual issues—from birth control and STD protection to sexual turn ons and turn offs—rethink what you are going to do sexually and with whom. You have to tell each other what your sexual values are and stand by your beliefs.

How sexually active should you be when dating, Michael? The ultimate guideline is that you should not do anything sexual that makes you or your partner feel uncomfortable, goes against your or her moral values or religious beliefs, or puts you and her at risk for a teen pregnancy, contracting AIDS, or other sexual diseases.

In my teen years making out and petting went like this: one partner (usually the guy) would go as far as he could until the other partner (the girl) told him to stop. Teens say that is still how it works today, though the girl is frequently the aggressive one. Often because of embarrassment or fear, saying "no" is difficult for both sexes.

How would you say "no" to a girl who is coming on too fast? First, you must be firm. If she has her hands on you, take her wrists in your hands and gently, but firmly remove her hands

from you. Still holding her wrists, look her straight in the eye
and say something like:

Stephanie,

I like you. I'm very turned on, but I am not going to
have sex with you. It's too easy for me to get you
pregnant—even with condoms, even when you are on
the pill. I am not going to mess up my life like that. I
want to be with you, but don't hassle me. I'm going to let
your wrists go now, and let's. . .(finish the sentence—go
back to the dance, game, concert, party, get something to
eat, etc.)

If she keeps hassling you, leave the situation. If you are going
together, break up. She doesn't respect you or herself. You deserve better. This can be hard to do. But it's better than her
telling you later on that she's pregnant.

Sex on television, in movies, and magazines gives many teens
the idea that if they like each other it's required they have sex.
If they were honest with each other, many guys and girls
would rather wait until they are older.

Before you begin dating or going with someone, know what
your sexual boundaries are. If a girl tries to cross those
boundaries, tell her no. You aren't comfortable going any further. Going further leads to having sex. Without birth control she can become pregnant even doing it one time.

You don't want to be a teen father. While your friends are
hanging out, you'll be working a job after school to pay child
support for your baby.

She does not want a baby in junior high or high school.
While her friends are out having fun, she'll have a 24-hour
baby sitting job staying home with her child.

It only takes one act of intercourse to become pregnant.

2,000 girls become pregnant daily in the United States.

Let's take relationships a step further. Say you are in junior high, middle school, or high school and are dating. You're probably playing the "Does she like me, do I like her?" game. You're learning all the rules—why we stay together and break up—and you're doing great! Then one of you wants to add intercourse to the relationship. Sex changes dating and the rules of dating. In my next letter we will explore some of the differences between what guys and girls think about sex and love.

> Take care of yourself,

> Mom

---

---

---

---

---

---

---

---

# LETTER 15

# WHAT Girls and Guys Think About Love and Sex

Dear Michael,

Girls and guys view sex and love differently because females and males are different. Our bodies are different. We have different hormones. We behave differently.

It's important for you to understand the differences between male and female behavior because it affects dating and relationships.

Generally, boys act masculine and girls act feminine. As young children, girls are more apt to reach for dolls, while boys are more apt to reach for trucks. Though males very capably raise children, the actual nurturing instinct to have children and a home usually surfaces earlier in females.

Males are usually factual versus emotional thinkers and females are the opposite. Being more emotional thinkers many girls see sex in dating as an act of intimacy in terms of like/love. Consequently a girl may become serious about a relationship before the guy is serious.

Being a factual thinker, you may see sex in dating as something that feels good rather than an expression of love. Not until a guy falls in love does he usually see sexual activity as an expression of love. You may fall in love as early as middle school or high school or not fall in love until your twenties or thirties.

The following are other differences and similarities between males and females.

* Females generally verbalize feelings more easily and more often than males. In relationships, girls often express their feelings regularly and they become frustrated when the guy is uncomfortable with "talking" about his feelings. There are also reverse situations where the guy shares all of his feelings and the girl isn't comfortable with intimacy.

* Most people don't like to be chased. If you come on to a girl too strongly, too fast, she may get scared and shut you out. Likewise if a guy knows a girl is chasing him, it usually makes him run even faster to escape.

* When you are dating, if you say "I love you," tell the girl what the "I love you" means. You may mean "I like you a lot," but your girlfriend may take it to mean "I love you forever."

When you date, ask what the "I love yous" you receive mean. "I love you" is often misunderstood because it can be said to express many different feelings. It may mean:

* I like you a whole lot (right now).

* I love you now when we're together but not forever. We're both in the eighth grade and forever is a long way off.

* I like you a whole lot (so let's keep going together and see if it turns into love).

- I love you as a friend (but not as someone to date).
- I love you as a person (but not as a date so let's break up).
- I love you so I can make out or have sex with you (I'm really only using you for sex).
- I love you forever.(This is the big I love you, usually reserved for monogamy or marriage).

The following summarizes some important points about love and sex.

- You will meet some girls who only want to date you for your car, your money, your status at school, or for sex. These girls will do anything and say anything, especially "I love you," in order to get you to buy them things, take them places, or have sex. If a girl only likes you for your body, car, or wallet—not for who you are as a person—she doesn't deserve you. Likewise, it's not right for you to tell a girl you like or love her in order to make out with her, have sex, or date her for status. Using each other for our own wants is cruel and selfish. Using people isn't what relationships and friendships are about.

- The majority of guys do not get serious about marriage until after high school—sometimes many years after high school. Girls sometimes think about marriage while still in high school. During high school you may become serious about a girl and she is not interested. She may change her mind after high school or she may not be the right person for you.

- When a girl falls for you, it can be as intense as when you fall for a girl. If you break up with a girl, it hurts her as much as it hurts you when a girl breaks up with you. Always be respectful of the other person's feelings during break-ups.

Michael, choose your friendships and dating relationships carefully. Listen to your heart, but use your brain!

With love and respect,

Mom

P.S. If puzzled by a relationship, refer back to this letter and Letters 13 and 14.

_____

_____

_____

_____

_____

_____

_____

_____

_____

_____

# Letter 16

# More About Love and Sex

Dear Michael,

What is sex? What is love? It's important you understand the difference—and when sex and love interconnect.

## Love

Whether platonic (non-sexual) or romantic (sexual), love is a deep caring for another person and sharing of yourself and your life with that person. You can love your friends and family (platonic love) and at the same time love someone you are dating (romantic love). In this letter I will concentrate on romantic love.

## Romantic Love

All romantic love begins as either a crush (infatuation), like/love or lust (intense sexual attraction towards another person). People fall in love in one of these ways.

### Crush (infatuation)

A crush occurs when you like a person, but you haven't told that person of your feelings. Usually a crush is fantasizing about a movie star, singer, teacher, or other person older than you who will not or can not return your feelings, and there is little chance the two of you will date. In seventh grade I had an intense crush on a sophomore in high school who never knew I existed. But I spent hours thinking about us being together. Have you had any crushes?

## Like/Love

Like is simply liking a person. You are attracted to a person's pleasing personality and looks. Like is the most stable of attractions and the one most likely to grow into love. Like is one of the foundations of a good relationship. Like is what you should strive for when dating. Have you had any "like" relationships yet?

## Lust

Lust is the trickiest of attractions because lust is a purely physical and sexual attraction. A girl may have the greatest body or sexiest smile you've ever seen. You want her. You don't know why you are obsessively attracted to this person, but your body is telling your brain that you want this girl. Never mind that once you get to know her the two of you are incompatible, or she's using you. Lust is a giddy, energy charged sexual high that may happen many times throughout your life. Lust is dangerous.

Lust-only relationships don't last. Lust can easily trick you into sex without birth control. It can also trick you into a relationship where sex rather than mutual respect and caring dictates the relationship.

It's probable that during your life you will find yourself almost uncontrollably attracted to someone. To determine if you are in lust or like/love, take the Lust vs. Like/Love Quiz (p. 131). Check the statements that best describe your feelings about your relationship. Then use the scorecard on page 132 to evaluate your feelings.

---

## LUST VS. LIKE/LOVE QUIZ

### Check Your Answers

**It's Lust**

❑ Your date's "body" is the main attraction.

❑ Few qualities attract you to your date, though the ones that do may be strong.

❑ The relationship started in a matter of hours or days.

❑ Your interest in the relationship comes and goes. It's not consistent.

❑ The relationship's effect on your personality is destructive. You're moody and not yourself.

❑ You live in a one-person world. You worship your date, seeing her as faultless.

❑ Few or no friends approve of the relationship.

❑ Distance hurts the relationship—it withers or dies.

❑ Fights are frequent and severe.

❑ You speak in terms of I/me/my; she/her/hers; there is little feeling of being a couple.

❑ Your ego response is mainly selfish. "What do I get out of this relationship?"

❑ You're possessive, jealous —afraid that at any minute the relationship might end.

**It's Like/Love**

❑ Your date's personality and body attract you.

❑ Many or most of your date's qualities are attractive to you.

❑ The relationship develops over months or years.

❑ Your interest level in the relationship is consistent.

❑ The relationship is constructive; you're happy, calm, secure.

❑ You realistically see each other's faults, but like/love the person anyway.

❑ Most or all friends approve. You get along with each other's friends and parents.

❑ The relationship survives distance.

❑ Fights are not frequent, nor severe. Compromise for each other's feelings comes easily.

❑ You feel and think as a unit. You speak in terms of we/us/our relationship.

❑ Your ego response is unselfishness and caring for your girl.

❑ You're secure in the relationship. Possessiveness and jealousy are infrequent.

---

(Lust-vs.-Like Quiz compiled from SEX, LOVE OR INFATUATION, by Ray E. Short, copyright 1978, 1990, Augsburg Publishing House. Use by permission of Augsburg Fortress.)

---

### Lust vs. Like/Love Scorecard

**0 - 4 checked responses in Column 1**
The relationship has possibilities but you need more time.
Re-evaluate monthly.

**5 - 13 checked responses in Column 1**
It's probably lust. The relationship might turn into like/love
but it's doubtful.

**0 - 4 checked responses in Column 2**
This could be the beginning of a nice relationship but you
need more time. Re-evaluate monthly.

**5 - 13 checked responses in Column 2**
It's likely that this is genuine like. Take your relationship
slowly. There is still much to discover about each other.

Later on in the relationship, if you think the like is turning
into love, ask your girlfriend to take this test. See if she rates
a score similar to yours.

---

## Regarding High School Sex and Love Today, Teens Said:

- "Sex is short term."

- "Love is not just saying, 'I love you.' There's more to it.
  You have to have feelings for someone."

- "Love is enjoying being with a person whether you're
  having sex or not."

As you can see, love and sex are different. We've talked about
love; let's talk about sex.

Sex means different things depending on how the word is
used. Being sexual with someone can mean activity as simple

as holding hands and kissing, or it can mean making-out, heavy petting, intercourse, or oral-genital sex.

Having sex (making love, doing it, messing with) means having intercourse, the man's penis inside the woman's vagina. Sharing your body like that is the most intimate way for you to be close to someone. Emotionally, intercourse touches a deep part of your inner self. When two people give their bodies to each other they become vulnerable to each other. You lay open your soul to another person.

If two people have a loving, mutual commitment, having sex is wonderful and fun. It strengthens and nurtures a relationship. But when one person is using the other person for sex or one person is more committed to the relationship than the other person, the relationship will not last. That happens often in teen dating.

The sex drive is present in all people once they experience puberty. During puberty it's important that you begin forming personal beliefs about love and sex. Then in middle school or high school you'll be able to stand true to your personal standards in making sexual decisions.

Having sex is emotional and physical. Physically, intercourse releases sexual tension from sexual arousal. Some people only have sex for the physical rush. For them, there is no love involved.

Others have sex without love because they don't know how to love. Some people have been hurt by love and stuffed their feelings. Until they risk loving again, they experience sex only on a physical level.

Still others, such as rapists, sexual abusers, and child molesters use sex for power, control, or punishment. They are physically or mentally sick—and many are acting out abuse they suffered as children.

Intercourse between two people who care for each other can be exciting and fun. But intercourse where one person is pressuring the other or using her or him for sex, hurts the person being used. Sex just for sex is superficial and not emotionally satisfying.

Intercourse shouldn't be added to any relationship until:

- the couple has had plenty of time to get to know each other (at least a year),

- they are mature enough to use contraceptives and STD protection,

- they are mature enough to handle the new emotions intercourse will bring to the relationship, and

- they are not going against their moral or religious beliefs.

Liking or loving someone does not mean you must have sex with that person. There are many non-sexual ways for couples to be close to each other.

- Going to the movies
- Sitting and talking to each other
- Writing letters to each other
- Going dancing
- Cooking dinner for each other
- Going to the zoo together
- Feeding the ducks at the park
- Jogging or bicycling together
- Touring a museum hand in hand
- Going to sporting events, concerts, or plays
- Picnicking in the park
- Riding horses

+ Boating, sailing, or skiing together

+ Playing miniature golf, basketball, or bowling together

+ Skating, ice skating, skiing, or sledding together

+ Racing go-carts

+ Doing volunteer work together

+ Doing homework together

Contrary to what movies and books often portray, dating does not mean immediately having sex. However, many people today throw intercourse into relationships before they know each other well enough to be intimate.

Once you share your bodies with each other, the dynamics of the relationship change. You expect more out of each other. You or your partner may be more protective, jealous, even obsessive. You or she may demand regular reassurances that the relationship is solid and going somewhere.

Sometimes in teen relationships the guy can handle the intimacy but his girlfriend can't or his girlfriend can handle the intimacy but he can't. Either way, the relationship breaks up.

Because teen dating is generally short-term dating (weeks or months) adding sex to these relationships increases the pain when you break up. Sure you may enjoy touching and making out, but I'd like you to save intercourse for your twenties when you have more experience with relationships and you are into long-term relationships.

Many guys have no idea what is pleasurable to the female during intercourse. They may have an orgasm, but they don't know how to help a girl have an orgasm. They haven't learned how the female clitoris functions. If that is so, sex is a big let down for the girl, while the guy wants more sex.

One way you can release sexual tension when you are sexually excited is to masturbate. Ninety percent of people surveyed said they masturbate. However, masturbation/self-touching is a topic that embarrasses some people. Granted, self-touching isn't something you talk about at the dinner table, but it is a perfectly healthy private activity.

Some teens think that only lesbians and gays masturbate, and that masturbating means they're homosexual. Another rumor claims that people only masturbate because they're not having sex. Both of these myths are false.

Self-touching is about being comfortable with your body. You're not gay if you touch yourself. For teen couples considering intercourse, bringing each other to orgasm through partner stimulation is a much safer way to enjoy sexual intimacy than risking pregnancy and STDs.

If you don't feel comfortable masturbating, that's okay too. Some people don't believe in self-touching. They exercise or take cold showers to release sexual tension. You're normal whether you do or don't masturbate.

Will you ever make mistakes dating, Michael? Will you think a girl is fine and she turns out to be a bad date? Will you ever be lured into a situation that compromises your sexual values? It's possible.

Your dad told me that he was once at a party and this girl needed a ride home. They got in the car and she started attacking him—kissing him, groping him, and trying to take off his clothes. He liked the girl, but he did not want to have sex with her because she was high and way out of control. He said he had to scream at her to get her to stop. She calmed down, but he said he could just imagine them having sex and the next day her accusing him of rape.

Everyone makes mistakes, Michael. What is important is whether or not we learn from our mistakes. I still remember my first boyfriend; your dad remembers his first girlfriend.

Parents were teens once, too. We know all about making-out and having sex and how confusing dating can sometimes be. If you ever get into a sexual situation that's moving too fast for you, your dad and I are here if you need to talk. Maybe it's a girl who's coming on too strong, too fast. Maybe you and a girl really like each other, the making out has become intense, and you're nervous because the next step looks like intercourse. Maybe you've just had your first sexual experience, it's messing up your head and you need to talk.

Your dad and I couldn't talk to our parents about sexual issues when we were teens. Our folks were uncomfortable talking about sex. I hope it will be different for you, but if you don't feel comfortable talking to us, talk with a school counselor or other adult you trust.

I think you'll find my next letter interesting. It deals with having sex and how to know when it's right for you.

Here's to knowing the difference between love and sex,

Mom

_____

_____

_____

_____

_____

_____

_____

_____

_____

_____

# LETTER 17

## INTERCOURSE
## WHEN IS IT RIGHT FOR YOU?

Dear Michael,

We're tackling a serious question, here. This letter gives you examples of why teen intercourse is not a good idea. Ultimately, you are the one who makes the decision.

I personally don't believe that having sex enhances any teen or adult relationship until the couple is committed to each other for the long-term and they understand the difference between love and sex.

When teens have sex, the emotional stress of new intimacy and the reality of possible pregnancy are important issues. Current statistics show that many teens aren't using birth control and STD protection, or they aren't using it correctly or regularly.

**Each day in the United States one out of every ten teenage girls become pregnant—2,000 daily! Nine out of ten guys leave their pregnant girlfriends.**

You probably know of kids in your school who are getting into sex too fast. Because of peer pressure, it's important from junior high on to be clear with yourself about teen intercourse. I personally hope you won't have sex as a young teen and that you won't ever have casual sex. I say this out of concern that your teens and twenties be free of pregnancy, STDs, and stressful relationships.

Here are comments from some high school males about having sex:

+ Don't have sex until you and your partner are both ready. It's not right to date girls just to see if you can have sex with them. Having sex with a lot of girls doesn't make you cool, it just means you are taking your chances with STDs.

+ Make sure every move is approved by the woman. Don't get it in your head that every time you go out on a date that will include sex. That has got to be the most false thing in males' heads today.

+ Treat your girlfriend with kindness and respect. Don't cheat, and if you are having sex, wear a condom.

+ Make sure you are 100% ready to have sex before you do, and make sure you really love that person.

The bottom line is:

+ Never have sex without a condom.

+ Never let yourself be pressured into having sex.

+ Don't use drinking or drugs as a source of courage to talk yourself into having sex before you're ready.

I hope when you're an adult that you find a special woman with whom you can have a wonderful lifetime relationship. Just as building a good relationship takes time, being sexually comfortable with someone takes time. One teen put it this way. "As for girls in general, you will break up and go out and then break up and go out and it may be a pain in the butt, but you can have good relationships so don't give up."

The majority of people do not have great first sexual experiences. For some guys, the first experience of having sex is full of anxiety. Since you've never done it before, you are not sure if you are doing it right. If the girl's vagina has not lubricated, having sex can be painful for both of you. The penis needs lubrication from the vaginal walls to slide into the vagina. A couple should know each other well and be relaxed with each other. Couples should be able to talk about their sexual likes and dislikes and feel comfortable enough with each other to be honest. That's why it is important not to rush sex in a relationship. Wait until you find that special relationship.

Some first sexual experiences of young people involve abuse. They are molested or raped by family members, acquaintances, or friends. Sexual abuse and rape are crimes. If you know anyone in that situation, have them read my letter on sexual abuse and talk to a school nurse, counselor, or the local county health department immediately.

All the males interviewed agreed that having sex changes a relationship. If you really care about a girl, you'll wait until she is ready, and you won't hassle her. Likewise she won't hassle you until you are ready.

Once you have sex and if it is a pleasurable experience, you will probably want to continue having sex. Sexual arousal is extremely powerful. You could begin to feel as though every girl you date is a candidate for sex. The truth is they are not. Michael, there will probably be only one or two women in your lifetime with whom you could develop a lasting relationship. Once you've had sex with someone your relationship will be more complicated and breaking up more difficult.

If you do end up having intercourse as a teen, use condoms every time and prepare yourself for the intimacy. Consider the following questions before adding intercourse to a relationship.

+ Will the relationship become nothing but sex?

+ Will sex help our relationship or destroy it?

+ What if my girlfriend becomes pregnant? Am I ready to be a teen dad?

+ Do I have the money to raise a child?

+ Would my girlfriend be a caring, responsible mom?

+ How many after high school plans (college, job, travel) will I have to postpone or change due to teen pregnancy or early marriage?

Sex complicates relationships. If you were involved sexually with a girl, how would you talk to each other about these concerns?

*Mom,*

*I like the idea of waiting to have sex until I'm in a serious relationship, but there is a lot of peer pressure. For guys it's a macho thing.*

To stand up for yourself takes courage, guts, and not being afraid to be your own person. If people hassle you, walk away. Or look them in the eye and say, "Why do you even care about my sex life? You're the one who should be worrying about AIDS." When you can stand up to peer pressure you are becoming a man.

Michael, you are right for standing firm in your beliefs. Choose friends who like you for you and not for your decision as to when you have sex.

Will you have sex as a teen, Michael? If you believe that intimacy should be saved for marriage, you'll wait to have sex until you find the girl you want to spend your life with. There is nothing wrong with waiting until you are married or engaged.

I hope you will wait until your twenties when you've had some experience with relationships. If you wait, you'll be more knowledgeable about using condoms and using them correctly. You'll be better prepared to handle the emotional feelings of having sex. You'll also be more likely to recognize when a girl genuinely cares about you or she's using you.

In addition to waiting until you've had some experience with relationships, there are also these concerns to consider:

* Teen Fatherhood. The objective of high school is to prepare you for living on your own. If you want to have a car, clothes, an apartment—you need to graduate and obtain some type of job training (technical school, military, college, apprenticeship) after high school. Being a teen father means eighteen years of child support payments. Being a teen father makes life complicated.

* AIDS will kill you. Because of AIDS you need to know the girl you are dating and her background. AIDS has been transmitted to the teen population. It's suspected that thousands of teens are now carrying the virus.

* STDs are rampant among teens. Often, teens have sex and never ask each other about their sexual histories. When you have sex with a girl without using condoms, you're having sex with everyone she has ever previously had sex with. This is how STDs, including AIDS, are transmitted.

* When a couple jumps into sex too soon, it's easy to become so wrapped up in each other that you drop out of life, your grades fall, and you neglect your friends. Nationwide, only one percent of high school dating relationships turn into life-long commitments.

- Having pre-marital sex would violate your moral and/or religious beliefs.

See page 145 for a summary of dumb and good reasons for having sex. You can probably add some of your own reasons to the list.

## You're Not Yet Ready for Sex

Most people are really not ready to handle intercourse until after high school. The following may be helpful to you in postponing sex until you're ready.

Respect Yourself. Don't play the macho game. Be a real man who cares about relationships.

Don't give in to any girl who wants sex. One of three things may happen:

1) she'll tell you she is using birth control when she is not *(Remember:* protecting yourself against an unwanted pregnancy and STDs is *your* responsibility)

2) she'll get possessive,

3) she'll use you and then talk about you.

Only when a couple has a long-term, stable relationship and it's a mutual agreement between the couple should intercourse be added.

- Limit time alone with your girlfriend if you're both not ready for sex but you don't have much will power when you're horny.

- Don't drink or do drugs. Alcohol and drugs distort your thinking and you can find yourself having sex without condoms. When you are high, you do stupid things that put you at risk for AIDS and other STDs and teen fatherhood.

## Dumb Reasons to Have Sex

1. Peer pressure. So what if your friends are having sex. You control when the time is right for you. If they tease you or pressure you, they're not real friends.

2. Curiosity; to see what it's like. With pregnancy, AIDS, and other STD health risks, this is not safe.

3. One-night stand. you meet a girl at a party. You like her, but you don't know her. With AIDS and STDs, casual sex is out. Don't risk it.

4. You think it will make you grown-up. It won't. Sex immediately complicates your life.

5. You're pressured into sex by a girlfriend. You think by doing it, you will keep or catch her. This plan usually backfires.

6. You let drinking or drugs be your excuse.

7. You do it to be popular. This backfires and gives you a reputation.

8. You do it to defy your parents or get their attention.

9. Confusing sex for love. You want to be loved so you substitute sex for love.

## Good Reasons to Have Sex

1. You're married, and sex with your wife is an expression of love.

2. You're in a long-term committed relationship. You want to share your love with each other, and. . .

a. You're not going against your moral or religious beliefs.

b. You know each other to be free of AIDS and STDs.

c. You feel that you are both mature enough to handle the intimacy of sex. You've talked to each other about having sex. You know that adding intimacy to your relationship will affect your relationship in new ways.

d. You reach a mutual agreement to have intercourse.

e. You've decided on and purchased the type of birth control you'll use.

You are a sexual person. Your hormones can be so active you may feel like your insides are bouncing off the walls. Your sexuality is a real part of you. Relationships are a part of growing up. But having sex before you and your partner are mature enough to handle the intimacy only causes hurt.

At what age will you have intercourse? It's different for everyone. When you become sexually active depends on your moral beliefs and values. You should not have sex until you're mature enough to use condoms and you can handle the emotional part of sex in a relationship.

When you have intercourse is your decision. If you feel that religiously or morally sex should be saved for marriage, then wait until you're married. If you have sex as a teen, you need to be responsible about birth control, and prepare yourself emotionally for the new feelings sex will bring to your relationships.

After reading this letter, you'll know that the decisions you make about sex will affect your life in many ways. I know you care about yourself. I know you'll be responsible.

Choose well. Be sure before you jump.

Mom

_____

_____

_____

_____

_____

_____

_____

_____

# LETTER 18

# SEXUAL DISEASES

Dear Michael,

Sexually transmitted diseases and AIDS are nothing to mess around with. STDs can make you sterile (unable to have children). AIDS will kill you: currently there is no cure. In 1992 the fastest growing number of HIV-positive cases—the virus that causes AIDS—was among teens. In your school, one out of three sexually active teens will contract an STD each year. This could be you or one of your friends. Here is one high school senior's story.

> Since my junior summer I've had sex with three girls—each during the time we were going together. I knew two of them weren't virgins, but none of our crowd could have STDs. And they were on the pill, so I didn't use condoms. Last month I started having a pus-like, yellowish discharge from my penis and burning when I peed. I went to the county health clinic and found out I had gonorrhea. The doctor gave me some antibiotics to cure it, but I was more than a little embarrassed, and I had to tell all three girls that they should get checked—that was a big hassle. Now I think twice before I add sex to relationships. If I do have sex, I always wear a condom.

Some STDs occur only through intercourse, but a number of STDs can also be transmitted through heavy petting and oral-genital sex. Obviously, the surest way to avoid STDs is to be abstinent—postpone having sex until you find your life partner. If this is not what you choose, you will have to protect yourself against STDs and AIDS in all sexual relationships.

Some warning signs of an STD may be:

- Unusual discharge from the penis

- Itching, burning, sores, rashes, or redness on the penis

- Pain or tenderness in the genital area or lower abdomen

- Pain or burning feeling when urinating; frequent urination

If you ever have any of these symptoms, see a doctor immediately.

Comments of Teen Males on Condoms, AIDS, and STDs

- "Always use a jimmy and don't be stupid and go sleeping around."

- "Don't let peer pressure lead you into something bad. Stay away from prostitutes. Wear condoms and be safe. Go get checked right away if you think you may have a sexual disease."

- "If you do have sex, always, and I repeat, always, use a condom. They are not 100% effective in blocking AIDS but they are better than nothing at all."

## Protect Your Body From STDs

Always carry and use condoms. Never let down your guard, "oh this one time won't matter."

Never have sex with a person you suspect isn't practicing safe sex (always using condoms).

Use a new condom for each act of intercourse. Condoms should never be reused. Pre-lubricated condoms with nonoxynol 9 currently offer the best protection and can be bought at any discount store, pharmacy, or convenience store. County health departments usually have free or inexpensive condoms. If you're embarrassed, go with a friend and purchase them together.

**Always use latex condoms pre-lubricated with nonoxynol 9, the spermicide that kills the AIDS virus and protects against pregnancy.**

If it doesn't say pre-lubricated on the package, don't buy that kind. The pre-lubricated latex condoms are a little more expensive than the non-lubricated, but when your life is on the line, spend the extra dollar.

## Talk frankly with your sexual partner about STD protection before you have sex

"Tara, I like you and this relationship. If we are going to have sex, I insist on a condom every time. Condoms are for protecting both of us. *No condom, no sex.*" You control the situation.

## Look before you love

Any sore, rash, or discharge your partner has may be a symptom of an STD. If you suspect anything, do not have sex. Do not engage in any heavy petting. Do not engage in oral-genital sex.

## Postpone having sex until you're ready and then, be choosy about sexual partners

Although condoms are the best protection other than abstinence, they are not 100% effective. Our sex drive is very powerful. Once you have sex, it's easy to add sex to every relationship. People who wait until their twenties to add sex to relationships are more apt to use STD protection properly and regularly.

Below are listed the ten most common Sexual Transmitted Diseases (STDs) affecting both males and females. There are also other less well known but equally dangerous STDs.

## Ten Most Common STDs— Affecting Both Males And Females

### AIDS (HIV virus)

*Increasing among heterosexuals, especially teens.*

Spread through oral-genital sex or anal or vaginal intercourse.

Symptoms: No early symptoms; later swollen glands, fever, diarrhea, night sweats, weight loss and fatigue.

Treatment: No cure. Early testing recommended, medications help retard onset of full AIDS.

Damage: Eventually death.

### CHANCROID

*More common in warm climates than cold.*

Spread by skin to skin contact.

Symptoms: Herpes-like sores, or ragged-edged pimples, or bright red blisters, on genitals or elsewhere on body.

Treatment: Antibiotics.

Damage: Open sores on genitals make it easy to pick up the HIV virus and other STDs.

### CHLAMYDIA (NGU in men)

*Fastest spreading STD in U.S. among fifteen to twenty-five year olds.*

Spread through intercourse and close sexual contact.

Symptoms: Called the "silent" STD, because there may be no initial symptoms until infection has began to damage reproductive system. Later painful urination, discharge in men; pelvic pain, itching, discharge, bleeding between periods in women.

Treatment: Antibiotics.

Damage: Causes sterility, ectopic pregnancies (outside the uterus usually in the fallopian tubes).

### GENITAL WARTS (HPV, Human Papilloma Virus)

*750,000 new cases a year, teens very susceptible.*

Spread through intercourse or oral sex.

Symptoms: One to three months after contact, very tiny flat, or cauliflower-like bumps appear inside/outside genitals.

Treatment: Warts frozen off or burned off with laser or electric needle.

Damage: Risk of genital cancer.

# Ten Most Common STDs (continued)

**GONORRHEA (clap dose, drip)**
*1-2 million cases a year, mostly people under twenty-five-years-old.*
Spread through intercourse, heavy petting if genitals touch.
Symptoms: frequent painful urination, discharge—sometimes no symptoms.
Treatment: Antibiotics.
Damage: Sterility, arthritis.

**HEPATITIS (Type B)**
*Very Common. Type B which is sexually-transmitted is the most dangerous.*
Spread by sexual contact, uncleanliness.
Symptoms: Dark urine, yellow eyes, tenderness in liver area, also flu like symptoms.
Treatment: Bed rest. Weeks, months to recover.
Prevention: Hepatitis vaccine, as a child or adult, usually available at county health department.

**HERPES SIMPLEX VIRUS-II (genital herpes)**
*500,000 to one million new cases each year.*
Highly contagious, spread by sexual contact, genitals and mouth.
Symptoms: Painful blister-like sores on genitals.
Treatment: Acyclovir eases pain, shortens attacks, but there is no cure.
Damage: Once contracted virus lives in body forever, and sores reoccur when person under stress. Sores painful, can cause blindness in babies of mothers who have active herpes. Uninfected sex partners are always at risk.
Note: Cold sores—herpes simplex-I is not genital herpes-simplex-II.

**PUBIC LICE (crabs) and SCABIES**
*Common in crowded living spaces.*
Highly contagious, spread mostly by sexual contact, close physical contact, contaminated towels, toilet seats, bedding, clothing.
Symptoms: Lice live in pubic hair; mites (scabies) burrow under skin. Severe itching, reddish zigzag furrows under skin.
Treatment: Creams, lotions and shampoo. Keep clean, bathe/shower daily.
Damage: Lice can carry other diseases.

**SYPHILIS (Syph, Pox, Bad Blood)**
*Infection rate at highest level in forty years.*
Spread by direct contact, usually sexual intercourse.
Symptoms: Painless red sores on genitals. Sores disappear, but disease remains in body to reoccur again.
Treatment: Penicillin or other antibiotics.
Damage: If not treated, syphilis can cause paralysis, dementia and death. Sores make it easier to contract AIDS.

**TRICHOMONIASIS (Trich)**
*Caused by tiny parasites that live in moist places in body. Common STD, but prompt treatment cures.*
Spread by sexual contact, shared damp wash clothes and towels, shared swimming suits.
Symptoms: Discharge with bad odor, frequent, painful urination.
Treatment: Best treatment is prevention. Wear cotton underwear, use condoms and spermicidal foam.

Michael, we only receive one body. It has to last us our entire lives—from birth on.

* Use pre-lubricated condoms with nonoxynol 9 spermicide every time you have sex.

* Get checked for STDs once a year at the health clinic or immediately if you have any symptoms.

* When you find a marriage or life partner, if neither of you are virgins, before having sex and/or marrying, each of you get tested for AIDS and other STDs.

Protect your body at all costs. Never let sexually transmitted diseases get control.

      With love,
      Mom

_____

_____

_____

_____

_____

_____

_____

# LETTER 19

# BIRTH CONTROL

Dear Michael,

In Letter 18, I discussed what you should consider before deciding to have sex. I also told you that I hope you wait until after high school. Whether teens are abstinent (not having sex) or sexually active, they should be familiar with birth control and the importance of using contraceptives. Anything less than using contraceptives every time, no exceptions, is like playing Russian roulette.

Birth control information is so important because of the increasing number of teen pregnancies that shouldn't be happening. I'll give you some general information about birth control and then discuss in detail each of the available contraceptives and effectiveness rates. There is a lot to cover. Let's get started.

When the time comes that you want to add sex to a relationship, you and your partner need to talk about birth control and what will work best for you as a couple. It's important that you know the different types of birth control available to females. Then you'll be able to talk to your partner about what birth control you and she will use—the condom and the pill, the condom and foam, or a combination of other methods.

If you didn't take a sexuality education class in school, you can take family planning classes for young couples from a county health clinic. If your partner won't go to the birth control class, ask yourself if she is as committed to the relationship as she says. Birth control is the responsibility of both partners.

### How do my partner and I get contraceptives?

When the time comes that you add sex to a relationship, you can make an appointment with our family doctor if that feels comfortable to you. If not, there are other alternatives such as health clinics. You can find them listed in the phone book or ask your friends.

### Many clinics offer free contraceptives

Clinics take after school appointments. Some even have evening and Saturday hours. The health clinic accepts all ages, and your visit is strictly confidential. If a clinic is not available in our town, you may have to drive to a neighboring town or county for services.

Contraceptives for females, such as the pill, Norplant, Depo-Provera, and the diaphragm require a visit to a clinic or family doctor.

The only 100% effective method of not creating a pregnancy is abstinence (not having sex). If that is not what you choose, you and your partner need contraceptives.

### What if I'm not sure that a clinic assures confidentiality?

When you call for an appointment, ask the clinic if they ensure confidentiality. Be sure to get the name of the person you talked to. If they say yes, by law your visit is confidential.

# Can I buy non-prescription birth control at a store without going to a clinic?

Yes, you can buy non-prescription contraceptives such as condoms and foams, but they are only effective against pregnancy when a couple uses them correctly. It's important to learn about birth control from the health clinic, school nurse, or through your school's sexuality education classes before purchasing condoms, foams, or other non-prescription forms.

# How do I get to the clinic to get condoms if I can't drive?

Ask a friend to take you, or you can ask me. In the city, you can take the bus.

# Should my girlfriend go to the clinic also?

Yes! Birth control is the responsibility of both the man and the woman. Condoms are not 100% effective, so your partner needs to use effective birth control along with the condom.

Males who are sexually active also need to visit the clinic for STD checks between relationships. In order for you to have children someday, your reproductive system must be kept infection free.

Once a female becomes sexually active, it's essential that she have a yearly pelvic exam and pap smear to keep her free from disease. If your partner and you are mature enough to have sex, she is mature enough to have an annual exam. Young women who aren't sexually active usually don't need annual exams until they reach age eighteen.

If your girlfriend is squeamish about having a yearly exam, please stress to her the importance of yearly exams. Offer to go with her to the clinic. Today, couples attend family planning clinics together.

## What will happen when I go to a family planning clinic or county health clinic?

If you want condoms, you can probably walk in anytime during business hours, ask for a supply of condoms and leave, no questions asked.

If you accompany your girlfriend to her annual exam or for birth control classes, usually a nurse or receptionist will greet you at a check-in desk. You will be asked to fill out a form asking for your name, birth date, health status, and other important information. The information is confidential—no one will know that you are a clinic patient.

If it's your first visit, you and your girlfriend will attend an initial family planning class covering contraceptives, STDs, and essential body care. There will be many other young men and women visiting the clinic too.

## How much does an exam and birth control cost?

Often, condoms are free. Other contraceptive costs vary depending on the type. Fees at county and Planned Parenthood clinics are based on your income. Also, purchasing supplies month by month can ease the expense by spreading the cost over time. At most clinics, even if you don't have money, you can get birth control.

Michael, the following information gives you contraceptive effectiveness rates and details the various methods. Before you become sexually active, read and reread this information carefully.

# BIRTH CONTROL CHART
## In order of effectiveness re: typical use

**Abstinence** (not having intercourse)—100% effective. Of 100 girls, zero will become pregnant.

**Sterilization** (surgical vasectomy—males, tubal ligation—females)—100% effective. A permanent birth control method for persons who have decided they absolutely do not desire any more children.

**Norplant®,** (five-year contraceptive implant). Studies show effectiveness greater than the pill; 100 girl comparison not available.

**Depo-Provera®,** (the three-month shot). Studies show effectiveness greater than the pill; 100 girl comparison not available.

**The pill** (oral contraceptive)—97% effective. Of 100 girls, three may become pregnant during first year of use. Women who take the pill at the same time daily, have less than a one percent chance of becoming pregnant.

**Male condom**—88% effective—more effective with foam. Of 100 girls, twelve may become pregnant during first year of use.

**Female condom** -two types now available. 100 girl comparison not available.

**Diaphragm/Cervical Cap with Spermicidal Jelly**—82% effective. Of 100 girls, eighteen may become pregnant during first year of use. High ineffectiveness rating may reflect incorrect usage.

**VCF, Vaginal Contraceptive Film**—effectiveness comparable to that of other spermicides—foams, jellies, suppositories, 100 girl comparison not available.

**Suppositories/Foam/Jellies**—79% effective. Of 100 girls, twenty-one may become pregnant during first year of use.

**IUD** —a prescription contraceptive that only women who have had a child and who are in a monogamous relationship may use. Of 100 women three may become pregnant during first year of use.

**Fertility Awareness Method W/Abstinence**—76% effective. Of 100 girls, twenty-four may become pregnant during first year of use. This is an involved and somewhat complicated method of charting ovulation, this birth control method is not recommended for young, unmarried women.

Information compiled in part from: J. Trussell, R.A. Hatcher, W. Cates, F.H. Stewart, and K. Kost, "Contraceptive Failures in the United States: an Update," *Studies in Family Planning* 21 (1), 1990.)

## Male Birth Control

### Abstinence—100% effective

Abstinence (not having intercourse) is the only 100% effective way of not getting someone pregnant. Kissing, hugging, caressing, and holding hands are ways to show your love for each other without having sex. *Note:* If a couple is into heavy making out and the male ejaculates, extreme care must be taken so that semen does not get anywhere near the girl's vagina. Sperm close enough to the vaginal opening can find their way into the vagina.

*Advantages:* No chance of pregnancy. Relationship is easier and less complicated. You don't have to hassle with the stress intercourse puts on a relationship.

*Possible Problems:* Couples who have gone together for a long time and are into heavy making out have to use strong will power to resist not having sex.

### Condom—88% effective for birth control, 98% effective against STDs

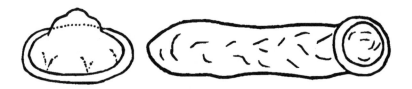

### Rolled-up and Unrolled Condom

Second to abstinence in effective birth control is the condom. The condom (rubber, jimmy, prophylactic) is a sheath of strong, thin latex (rubber) that you roll onto your erect penis before intercourse. If the condom does not have a pre-molded reservoir at the end to contain the semen after ejaculation, you must leave slack in the end of the condom to hold the semen. Some condoms are made with reservoirs, others are not. Condoms are so thin that neither male or female should sense any loss of feeling when using them.

Six Steps of Using a Condom

1) Open the packet.

2) Grasping the rolled-up condom with both hands, put it on the end of the erect penis. If the condom doesn't have a pre-molded reservoir (small oval shape on the end of the condom), leave some room at the tip of the condom to catch the semen.

3) Continue to slowly slide the condom onto the penis. It will unroll until it is all the way on.

4) After intercourse, put your hand on the condom at the base of the penis so the condom doesn't slip off the penis and carefully remove the penis from the vagina.

5) Take both hands and roll the condom off the penis, staying away from the vagina so no sperm find their way into the vagina.

6) Throw the used condom away. Use a new condom for each act of intercourse.

Condoms are inexpensive, reliable, and easy to buy as a primary or secondary birth control method. They are available in a variety of colors and styles and can be bought without a prescription at almost any pharmacy, grocery store, or convenience store. Males can carry them in their wallets. Females can carry them in their purses.

*Caution*: When carrying condoms in your wallet, or your car throw away the condoms every two months and put in new ones. The wear and tear of the condom being in your wallet can cause the latex to crack or break, making them unsafe as birth control and STD protection.

*Never* use Vaseline® or any type of petroleum jelly as a vaginal lubricant with a condom. the Vaseline and jelly can dissolve the rubber. Water-based lubricants such as KY-jelly can be used safely—make sure the package states that the lubricant is water-based.

Young couples should not be embarrassed to use condoms. Couples can put the condom on the erect penis together as foreplay before intercourse. To be most effective in preventing pregnancy, condoms should be used with contraceptive foam (the female inserts foam into her vagina).

*Advantages:* Non-prescription, easy-to-buy, and inexpensive. Condoms are currently the most effective form of protection against STDs, other than abstinence.

*Possible Problems:* Semen can leak from the condom if the penis is not withdrawn properly from the vagina or rough handling of the condom tears the latex.

## Non-Contraceptives—do not prevent pregnancy

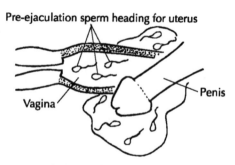

Pre-ejaculation sperm heading for uterus

Penis

Vagina

Withdrawal—0% effective

Males often think "I can withdraw the penis from the vagina before ejaculating." That doesn't matter. Pre-ejaculatory semen from the penis empties into the vagina before ejaculation. It doesn't matter if you withdraw before you ejaculate because sperm from the pre-ejaculatory semen is already in your partner's vagina, swimming upward to find an ovum. More teen pregnancies happen because people have heard withdrawal works. They are wrong.

## Drugs—0% effective

Marijuana, crack, cocaine, and acid do not affect male sperm development or a woman's ovulation cycle to the point that it prevents conception. A person high on drugs usually forgets all about birth control and STD protection.

## Douche—0% effective

Some females believe that douching after sex will kill the sperm. Douching *does not* kill sperm. In fact some researchers believe that the washing action actually propels the sperm into the cervix. If your partner says, "don't worry, I'll douche afterward," tell her *no sex* without a condom or other birth control. Tell her douching does not work.

## Abortion—not a contraceptive

Abortion is a medical procedure to terminate a pregnancy.

# Female Birth Control

Michael, it's important that you understand the different types of birth control for females. You need to know how they interact with your partner's body and what forms she may be able to use. As a couple you need to remind each other to remember to use birth control *every time* you have sex, *no exceptions*, unless you are married and planning a family.

## Not using birth control results in pregnancy

The three most effective forms of birth control currently available for females are Depo-Provera® (the shot), Norplant® (the five-year contraceptive implant), and oral contraceptives (the pill).

The pill, shot, or implant should not be used if your partner thinks she might be pregnant, has a history of blood clots or vein inflammation, high blood pressure, migraines, liver disease, unexplained vaginal bleeding, an abnormal growth, or cancer of the breast or uterus. A family history of diabetes or other generational diseases may also prohibit use.

## Norplant®—99% effective

The Norplant® implant is a five year low dose contraceptive consisting of six small, soft, flexible capsules placed under the skin of the upper arm. Norplant® works by continuously releasing levonorgestrel which inhibits ovulation. The implant

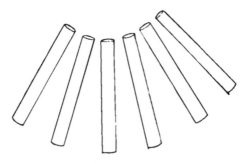

Norplant ® System

usually can't be seen unless the woman is very thin or muscular. Once they are in place, the capsules will not move around or break. If a woman desires pregnancy, the implant can be removed before the five-year time limit.

*Advantages*: Reliable pregnancy prevention for a five year period. Convenient, no hassles, constant protection.

*Possible Problems*: High initial cost, though very cost effective for five-year period. Must be implanted by a health care provider. Placement and removal may leave small scar. In some women, side effects may be greater than if taking the pill. Side effects may include prolonged menstrual bleeding, unexpected bleeding, nervousness, enlargement of ovaries and/or fallopian tubes, acne, excessive growth of body hair, or hair loss.

Depo-Provera® (the shot)—used in some countries more than thirty years

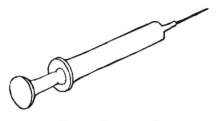

Depo-Provera®

Depo-Provera® (drug name: serile medroxyprogesterone acetate suspension, DMPA) is a contraceptive shot that is administered by a health care provider every three months. Your partner would get a shot four times a year. Depo-Provera® works by inhibiting follicle maturation and ovulation.

*Advantages*: Effectiveness rating greater than the pill. Constant three month protection. Cost spread out over a year in quarterly payments as opposed to the high initial cost of an implant.

*Possible Problems:* Your partner must remember to get her shot on time, or she will not be protected against pregnancy. Some people don't like shots. Side effects may include bloating, weight gain, headaches, depression, loss of interest in sex, and hair loss.

## The Pill (oral contraceptive) 97% effective

The Pill is still the most popular form of birth control for young women because:

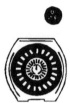

- the majority of females can take the Pill,

- it's easy and convenient to use, and

- it's initially less expensive than an implant.

*Caution your partner that she must take the pill every day at the same time.* Young women get pregnant frequently on the pill because they don't follow pill instructions.

Facts About the Pill

- To be effective the Pill must be taken the same time each day. Many women get pregnant by not taking their pill at a set time each day (example 7 a.m. daily or 5 p.m. daily). If your partner forgets a pill, she should call the clinic for further instructions and use another form of birth control if having sex. If she skips even one pill, she could easily become pregnant.

- Antibiotics and certain cough medicines can affect the Pill's effectiveness. At those times use a second form of birth control, such as a condom or foam spermicide to prevent pregnancy.

- When starting the Pill your partner must go through one month's pill prescription before the Pill begins to prevent conception.

- Although oral contraceptives are safe for many women, your partner may experience some mild side effects. If any of these symptoms become severe, call your clinic immediately.

- Oral contraceptives work by changing the level of hormones (progesterone, estrogen) in the body so your partner doesn't ovulate (produce a fertile egg) or build up the endometrium (lining of the uterus) in her uterus. By preventing these activities, no conception (pregnancy) occurs.

Pills come in a variety of hormonal types, levels, and monthly cycles. When taken correctly the Pill is 97% effective in preventing pregnancy. Oral contraceptives are safe for many women and may have fewer side effects than the implant or shot.

Your partner's doctor can determine if she can take the Pill and which Pill will suit her best. In certain cases the Pill has had medical value in reducing severe menstrual disorders, such as excessive menstrual bleeding, severe cramping, iron deficiency, pelvic inflammatory disease, non-cancerous breast tumors, ovarian cysts, and ovarian and endometrial cancer.

*Advantages*: When taken correctly, for most women it is an effective contraceptive with few side effects.

*Possible Problems*: Some women experience side effects, such as bloating, slight weight gain, headaches, depression, and mood swings. Your partner must remember to take the Pill daily.

## Diaphragm with Cream/Jelly—82% effective

The diaphragm is a soft rubber disk with a flexible rim and is used with contraceptive cream or jelly. The diaphragm comes in different sizes. It is a prescription contraceptive, and must be fitted by a doctor. To use the diaphragm, your partner squeezes the recommended amount of contraceptive cream into the diaphragm and inserts it into her vagina before intercourse so that it covers her cervix. The diaphragm stops the sperm from entering the cervix and the contraceptive cream kills the sperm.

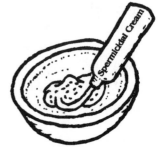

**Diaphragm with Spermicidal Cream**

To be effective, the diaphragm must be left in the vagina six to eight hours after your last intercourse before removing it. Diaphragms last anywhere from one to two years before needing replacement. Your partner should check her diaphragm frequently for tears or pin holes by holding it up to the light.

The diaphragm is a good choice for women who can't take the pill and for married couples. However, the diaphragm usually isn't prescribed for young unmarried women unless they are comfortable touching their bodies and are responsible about using birth control every time. Using a diaphragm means a commitment to using birth control every time.

*Advantages:* Once learned, insertion is easy and you and your partner can't feel the diaphragm. Many women feel that the diaphragm is not as messy as the condom. There are no side affects like those which can occur from the Pill.

*Possible Problems:* Even though most women have no side effects, some women may experience mild allergic reactions to the cream or jelly used with the diaphragm. The diaphragm can become dislodged during sex if the woman is on top or if she has a relaxed vagina as a result of childbirth. The diaphragm should be refitted after each childbirth or if a woman gains or loses more than fifteen to twenty pounds. If your partner experiences genital itching or irritation, unusual vaginal discharge, discomfort when the diaphragm is in place, any bladder infection, or pregnancy symptom, she should report it to her doctor immediately.

The diaphragm, pill, Norplant and Depo-Provera are prescription birth control that require your partner to have an exam at a health clinic or private doctor. You may wonder what exactly happens in an exam.

First a nurse will do a weight, urine, and blood check and then show your partner to a private room for a breast and pelvic exam, pap smear, and doctor consultation. Your partner can ask that you continue to be with her during this time, or she may feel comfortable having you remain in the waiting room until she's finished. You may date someone who would rather go the clinic for her annual exam by herself or with a girlfriend.

Usually, if a male doctor examines your partner at a health clinic, a female nurse will be in the room. If this is not so and your partner is uncomfortable, have her ask that a female nurse come in so the examination can continue.

If you are with your partner, the doctor may ask you to step outside for the examination and then have you return to discuss contraceptive use. This is simply doctor preference, so no one feels uncomfortable during the exam procedure.

## The Examination

Almost every young woman is concerned about her first breast and pelvic exam and pap smear. Your partner can calm herself by talking to herself, "I care about my body. Having an exam is part of keeping myself healthy. I will take deep breaths and relax. I'm having an exam because I care about my body." Females who are sexually active need a yearly breast and pelvic exam. Soon annual exams should become a simple routine.

There are normally three parts to the exam: breast exam, pelvic exam, and pap smear.

## Breast exam

During the breast exam the doctor checks the breasts for any abnormal lumps or cysts. Your partner should also perform this procedure on herself monthly right after her period. Many clinics have plastic examination cards she can place in the shower or near the bathtub as a monthly reminder. She can ask the doctor if these are available.

Breast cancer currently affects five to ten percent of all females. Your partner is at greater risk if there is a history of breast cancer in her family. Since early detection substantially increases the rate of recovery, monthly breast self exams and regular mammograms after age thirty-five should be a priority for all women.

## Pelvic exam

The pelvic exam consists of the doctor palpating the uterus and ovaries for any signs of abnormalities such as cysts or tumors.

## Pap smear

The pap smear consists of the doctor taking a speculum (a small metal or plastic appliance) to slightly open the vagina. A soft cotton swab is then used to gently scrape a few sample cells off the cervix. These cells are sent to a lab for detection of cervical cancer. Usually, if your partner doesn't hear from the clinic the test is negative (no cancer cells found). If the test is positive, the office will confidentially contact your partner through school or some other means. Having a positive test does not mean a person has cervical cancer.

Occasionally tests will turn up false positive. It does mean your partner will have to take a second test.

After completing the three exams, the doctor and your partner (and you if you are present) will discuss which contraceptives are best for her and your needs as a couple. Then the doctor will excuse her or himself to allow your partner to get dressed. At the health clinic your partner can usually pick up the birth control and condoms (for STD protection) before she leaves.

## Additional Birth Control

### VCF (Vaginal Contraceptive Film)
### used in Europe for eighteen years

Vaginal film is a thin, clear square of material containing a spermicide. The female puts the film over her middle finger and inserts her finger into her vagina so the film is placed on her cervix. Insertion takes practice; it's recommended that the woman practice inserting a few films before using one for intercourse. Her fingers must be completely dry before touching the film.

The film must be inserted not less than fifteen minutes and not more than one hour before intercourse. Once in the vagina the film dissolves into a thick gel that coats the cervical opening, killing sperm on contact. The body's natural fluids wash the gel away. A new gel must be used for each act of intercourse.

*Advantages:* Easy to use, few if any side effects and can be bought without a prescription.

*Possible Problems:* Must be used correctly to prevent pregnancy. Not 100 % effective. Not available in all stores at this time.

### Suppositories/Foams/Creams/Jellies—79% effective

These products are chemical substances inserted deep into the vagina before intercourse to kill the sperm while not harming vaginal tissue. Suppositories, foams, creams, and jellies are available in a variety of packages and under different names. If not used exactly as directed, these products may not form a good barrier to the uterus and pregnancy can result. Most brands are only effective at killing sperm one hour after insertion. To increase effectiveness these products should be used with a condom.

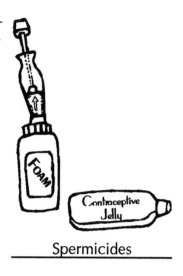

Spermicides

*Advantages:* These products can be bought by anyone at any age and they are fairly easy to use.

*Possible Problems:* Some women may experience genital irritation. Switching brands may help relieve the inflammation. Others may have an allergic reaction to any spermicide and can't use this form of contraception. Some women complain of leakage and messiness.

### Female condoms

There are now "female" condoms available that cover the inside of the vagina and outer labia. They are somewhat more complicated to use than the male condom and more expensive, but used correctly they can provide good protection. When the time comes that you and your partner need birth control, you can ask a doctor about condoms for females, and ask the doctor to explain their usage and effectiveness rating.

## Rhythm Method (fertility awareness with abstinence)— 76% effective

Fertility Awareness or Rhythm Method or Natural Family Planning is a form of birth control. To practice fertility awareness your partner must take her temperature and examine her vaginal mucus daily to chart her ovulation cycle. During her fertile time each month, the couple doesn't have sex. This method is not recommended for teens because of its low effectiveness rate.

*Advantages*: The rhythm method is natural; you aren't putting any kind of contraceptive in your body.

*Possible Problems*: Its low success rate means pregnancy is more probable. It requires continual tracking of the menstrual cycle. Like the pill and other methods there is no STD protection.

## Sterilization—100% effective

Today, sterilization (vasectomy for men, tubal ligation for women) is an increasingly popular form of permanent birth control for parents who have their families and don't desire more children or for couples or individuals who don't want to be parents.

Now that you've read about the different types of contraception, which ones do you like?

Michael, having sex is a mutual decision by a couple. What type of birth control you and your partner will use is a part of that decision. When the time comes, I know you will take care of yourself and your partner. When you need it, this chapter will be here for you to reread.

I love you,

Mom

_____

_____

_____

_____

_____

_____

_____

_____

_____

_____

_____

_____

# Letter 20

# Teen Pregnancy—Teen Fatherhood

Dear Michael,

Of all the letters in this book, this letter I wish I didn't have to write. I hate the fact that so many teens today have babies. As you become older, the desire to have sex can be intense. If you add intercourse to your relationships, what happens if a girl becomes pregnant? What do you do?

*If you have sex without birth control you will get a girl pregnant.*

## Teen Fatherhood and the Law

DNA testing is now generally accepted as a method of proving paternity (fatherhood). In addition, most states have been passing tougher child support laws. If you get a girl pregnant and she keeps the baby, you will likely be required to pay child support for the next eighteen years of your child's life. In our state:

- If you have a part time job, the state can garnish your wages for the child support.

- If you have a car, the state can make you sell the car to help pay hospital costs and child support.

- If you had college plans, the state can stipulate that you work a full-time day job instead. If you were looking at scholarships, most colleges do not award scholarships to teen dads.

- If you don't have a job, the state can make us (your parents) pay child support for your baby.

## Tragedies of Teen Pregnancy

Having a child is a serious commitment. It's a commitment you should never have to deal with in your teen years. However, some guys think getting a girl pregnant proves they are men. Some girls think they want to get pregnant to have someone to love them. A baby is not a way to *get* love, and getting someone pregnant doesn't make you a man.

A guy may think, if she gets pregnant, it's her problem. Wrong. A baby needs a mother and a father. Your child needs food, diapers, and health care. Equally important, a child needs the love and nurturing of a father and mother.

A teen parent has a twenty-four hour baby-sitting job that never goes away. You lose your friends, your fun, your freedom, your life. There is too much to learn, see, and do in high school to become teen parents.

I know when you make the decision to have sex you will use birth control. I know you won't let a girl trick you into a pregnancy. I hope you'll wait to add sex until after high school. I also know that sometimes contraceptives fail. I pray you never have to face a teen pregnancy.

### What Would Happen If You Got A Girl Pregnant?

The first thing I hope you'll do is tell me. An unplanned teen pregnancy is a traumatic, scary situation. Choosing how to handle an unplanned pregnancy is an important decision.

If you get a girl pregnant and she carries the pregnancy to term, you have an obligation to your son or daughter to support your child—that baby is made up of half of your genes. He or she is your child. But some guys are cowards and they run. The most cowardly thing a parent can do is run from his or her child.

According to *Family Planning Perspectives*, currently in the U.S., **each day 2,000 girls become pregnant and nine out of ten guys leave the pregnant mother.** But with new child support laws, deadbeat dads are being caught and made to pay up.

Would I be shocked when you first told me? Probably. I might ask: "Are you sure the girl is pregnant? Were you using birth control?" Please realize that these are normal parental first reactions because teen pregnancy is serious. Teen pregnancy will affect the guy and girl for the rest of their lives.

If you and the girl think she's pregnant, what happens next? If at all possible she should tell her parents. If she can't tell her parents, she needs to call the local family planning clinic immediately for help and she needs a pregnancy test to confirm the pregnancy.

If the test is positive, you and I should sit down and talk about her options so that you understand them. If she isn't comfortable telling her parents right away, she, you, and I can talk together.

Teen pregnancy is often a very sticky situation for the teen father. As a teen father you are subject to the particular laws of the state in which you live and in many states the final decision is up to the female because the pregnancy affects her body.

You may want the baby; she may want to give it up for adoption. She may want the baby; you may want adoption. She may want an abortion, and you don't, or vice versa. The girl may consider your feelings about how to handle the unplanned pregnancy, or she and/or her parents may not want you involved.

Even if state law doesn't require your monetary support, your child needs your support—your financial help and your love.

If there is any reason that you feel you might not be the father, we need to talk about that, too. In some states after the baby is born you can request a DNA test to establish whether or not you are the biological father.

Here are the most common pregnancy options:

Option 1: Have the baby and give it up for adoption.

If a couple isn't ready to become parents, carrying the pregnancy to term and putting the baby up for adoption is a good option. Adoption agencies have waiting lists of caring couples who desperately want children but can't have children of their own. These couples are screened for ability to love and nurture a child and provide a good home. In some adoption cases if the girl doesn't have insurance the adoptive parents will pay the hospital costs of the delivery.

Adoption laws and procedures vary in each state. Some states have open adoption where you can meet the adoptive parents and receive progress reports on the child. What do you think about the adoption option for teen parents?

Option 2: Have the baby and keep it.

Some teen mothers, after carrying their babies for nine months and seeing their babies, decide they can't give them up for adoption. But becoming parents is a lifetime commitment. Are you and your girlfriend ready to accept the responsibilities of parenthood?

State laws vary regarding child support and visitation. If the mother of your child is smart, she knows that a child needs both a mom and a dad. She and you can work out a parenting schedule. If the teen mom doesn't want you around, you may have to go to court to get visitation rights. Always remember, your child should be your primary concern. He or she needs and deserves your support and love, whether or not you and the child's mom stay together as a couple.

Becoming a teen parent means putting your child's needs first—feeding, diapers, and doctor visits. It means missing school activities and times with your friends to take care of your child.

Being a teen dad means maintaining your schooling to earn your high school diploma and working to pay for food and clothing for your child. It's almost impossible to get a good paying job without a diploma, and without a good paying job you can't support you and your child.

Many teen parents work hard to be good parents and good providers, but it's a tough life. For teens who can't handle the stress and responsibilities, grandparents often end up raising the kids. In abuse or neglect cases, a teen's children may be taken by child custody services.

If you and your girlfriend love each other, you may decide to have the baby, finish high school, and get married. When I was in high school, I knew a couple who kept their baby and married, and they are a happy family today. But, they happened to be part of the one percent of teens who find their marriage partners in high school. How do you feel about teens taking on the responsibilities of parenthood?

Option 3: Abortion—terminating the pregnancy

Michael, aborting a pregnancy is also an option that some females choose. A young woman may feel she could not be a mother at that time, or she could not handle the pregnancy.

Abortion is a touchy subject in America. People are divided by their moral and religious beliefs about abortion. Should

you ever have to deal with the abortion option in an unplanned pregnancy, this section gives you a brief overview
of the many sides of the abortion issue.

Some people have particular religious convictions about
abortion. They believe that "humanness" is present at the
moment of conception when the sperm fertilizes the ovum.
Therefore abortion, at any stage of pregnancy, is murder.

Other people don't believe that humanness begins at conception, so early abortions are permissible. They believe
that when the embryo begins developing into a fetus and
displays human features that "humanness" is present.

Still others believe that the zygote is a growing life from the
moment of conception. They would not choose abortion
for themselves, but they believe abortion is a private decision for each woman.

A few people don't view a pregnancy as a growing life. They
think abortion is fine, anytime.

Whose view is correct? I know that for myself and my
friends abortion is a deeply personal issue. The issue of terminating a pregnancy is an issue that will probably always
be debated.

For many years abortion was illegal in the United States. In
1973, the Supreme Court ruled that abortion was legal. In
1990, the Supreme Court ruled that states could set restrictions on abortion (such as 24 hour waiting periods and parental or judge's consent). Laws are constantly changing.
When you read this, abortion may or may not be restricted
in our state.

Legal abortion costs range from $200 for an early-term abor-
tion to over $2,000 for a late-term abortion. A woman can
contact her private doctor, county health clinic, or local
family planning clinic for more information. If abortion has
restrictions in one state, it may be possible to obtain an

abortion in a neighboring state. If someone chooses to abort a pregnancy, it is best done as early as possible in the pregnancy (within the first few weeks).

Medically speaking, abortion is a safe medical procedure when performed by a licensed doctor under sterile conditions. If performed before the twelfth week of pregnancy, abortion is physically less harmful to the female than carrying a pregnancy to term. Choosing to abort a pregnancy is not an easy decision, but in particular situations a woman may see it as her only choice.

If you don't believe in abortion, then the safest way to never deal with the abortion option is to not have sex until marriage—or if you do have sex, always use birth control. What are your feelings about abortion?

*Mom,*

>*I appreciate knowing you would be supportive if I ever got someone pregnant, but I have some friends who are afraid to talk to their parents. Other friends of mine could never tell their parents. Is there anything they can do?*

Good question, Michael. Telling parents about a pregnancy is a tough thing to do. If at all possible, teens should tell their parents. Parents may be shocked, hurt, or angry at first. But most parents really love their children and will want to help a daughter or son in this situation.

Teens who can't discuss the issue with their parents can call a family planning clinic or county health clinic. These clinics have professional, caring nurses and counselors who will help your friends consider their options. The important thing is to not delay calling someone for help.

Michael, as you can see, the choices one makes in a teen pregnancy aren't easy. The bottom line is that if you use birth control responsibly, you *probably* won't have to worry about an unplanned pregnancy. But if you make the choice to not add sex to high school relationships, you *definitely* won't have to worry about teen pregnancy.

I know you'll be responsible with your sexuality, Michael. I'm always here if you want to talk.

Mom

_____

_____

_____

_____

_____

_____

_____

_____

_____

# LETTER 21

# SEXUAL ABUSE

Dear Michael,

No one should ever force you to participate in any sexual activity or touch you sexually without your consent. This letter is about sexual abuse, incest, child molestation, and rape. Your body is yours. No human has sexual rights over another human. Likewise, you should never force anyone to have sex or touch them sexually without consent.

Both girls and guys are sexually abused. If you are ever a victim, tell me immediately. If for some reason you feel you can't tell me, tell the principal or counselor at your school or call our local county health or family planning clinic. If the first person you tell doesn't believe you, keep talking until someone does believe you.

Sexual abuse is a crime, Michael. It's a crime because one human is violating the body of another human. Sexual abuse causes psychological injury to its victims. Serious bodily injury including the transmission of STDs and AIDS also frequently occurs.

Sexual abuse is not new. Its destructiveness dates as far back as pre-biblical days. The difference is that today victims can get help; then they could not.

People sexually abuse and rape other people for many reasons. For most abusers, sexual abuse is a way to exert power or control over someone. The abuse isn't for sexual satisfaction. Some abusers are repeating the sexual, mental, or physical abuse they suffered as a child. Others are mentally ill.

Sexual abuse can range from a one-time incident of someone touching you sexually or forcing you to do something sexual, to a parent's repeated intercourse with her or his child. Sexual abuse can also be verbal abuse where the abuser manipulates the victim verbally, without physical touch. Sexual abuse is widespread. It's estimated that one out of three girls and one out of six boys will be sexually abused in some manner before their eighteenth birthday.

Michael, it is important that you know the types of sexual abuse, the effects of sexual abuse, and the ways you can lessen your chances of being sexually abused. Remember, both males and females can be and are sexually abused.

## Incest

Incest is defined as any sexual activity between members of an immediate family or step-family, other than normal wife-husband sexual relations. Incest can occur between a parent and child and between older and younger siblings.

Incest is serious. It's the type of sexual abuse most often kept secret or denied. Current statistics show that incest occurs in one out of every four families. The victims are usually threatened by their abuser or they feel ashamed so they never seek help.

Incest victims have confused feelings about love, sex, and self-worth. Unless treated, these feelings can haunt victims throughout their adult lives, affecting their relationships with a spouse, family, friends, and society.

*Note:* Brothers and sisters age five and under may play "doctor" or "mommy and daddy." While it should be discouraged when discovered, this type of sex play between young children is fairly common and normally is not incest. Being forced to have sex or play sex games with an older brother, sister, or relative is incest.

## Child Molestation

Child molestation is the same as incest, but the abuser is not necessarily an immediate family member. The abuser may be a relative—Cousin Jim, Grandpa Bill, Uncle George, or a family friend or business person—Neighbor Bob, Dentist John, Doctor Carl, or a complete stranger.

Though this type of abuse is called "child" molestation, the law covers any victim under age eighteen. For males, molestation may include touching of the genitals, anal intercourse, or being forced to perform fellatio (oral-genital sex).

One of my college friends told me about an abuse experience when he was in the sixth grade. At a weekend family reunion, an older cousin whom he didn't know well, forced my friend to perform oral sex on him. He never told his family and to this day that incident bothers him.

Incest and child molestation are crimes. Perpetrators (abusers) should not be allowed to continue these activities. When a victim (child or teen) reports an abuse, the victim needs counseling to heal from the negative psychological effects of the abuse. The abuser should be punished for the crime and get treatment for his or her sickness.

## Rape

Rape, in any form, is defined as a person forcing sexual intercourse on another person. In some states rape occurs when anyone under age fourteen has intercourse, even with joint consent. It is also rape if the person taken advantage of is mentally handicapped.

Rape happens most often to women, but too often men are also victims. You need to know how to avoid it ever happening to you—male to male. You also need to know how to make sure you never participate in rape or abuse or take the unnecessary risk of being accused of rape.

I know a man who, as a college student, was raped anally by another male. He never reported the rape because at the time he was too embarrassed. To this day, the incident still troubles him.

There are also documented court cases of females raping males, (at gunpoint, tying them up, etc.). Although this isn't an every day occurrence, it does happen.

## Acquaintance/Date Rape

In 60% of female rapes, the rapist is known by the victim— he is a casual acquaintance or she is dating him. I don't know if any organization has statistics for male acquaintance rape, but I would imagine the percentage to be similar.

Many acquaintance and date rapes go unreported. The victim often feels responsible for the rape thinking "I shouldn't have been in that situation in the first place" or "I was drinking and doing dumb things."

Humiliated and fearing punishment from parents, teen victims often never tell anyone about the rape. But victims should talk. Victims who can't confide in their family should tell a school counselor or someone at the local county health clinic.

If you should ever be raped or sexually abused in any way, I want to know about it. Any type of rape and even attempted rape is traumatic. It's important that you talk to a therapist so you can resolve the trauma and go on with life. It's also important for your health that you have an STD check, including testing for AIDS.

Whether it's a chance meeting, first date, or a long-term relationship, rape or abuse can happen. All too often male victims are so shaken by the abuse they won't seek help or press charges. They think, "I'm too embarrassed. I can't risk asking for help. My abuser will hurt me (or leave me) if I tell what happened."

Sexual assault is never the victim's fault, even if he was in the wrong place at the wrong time. Rape and abuse are crimes. If you are ever raped or sexually abused, seek help immediately.

To learn how to protect yourself from rape and sexual abuse, practice the following safe-guards.

## Protecting Yourself Against Incest, Sexual Abuse, and Rape

* Stay away from people you don't trust and those you feel uncomfortable being around. If someone repeatedly engages you in sexual talk, touches you, or brushes up against your body tell me, a teacher, school counselor, or social worker. We want to help you deal with that person.

* If confronted by an exhibitionist (flasher) keep your cool. Don't say anything. Turn away and walk to the nearest phone, dial 911, and report the incident. Flashers are normally harmless, but don't take chances. Never provoke one.

* If someone—a relative, friend, acquaintance, or stranger tries to abuse you sexually, there are three steps to follow: (1) Say "No!" (2) Get away. (3) Tell someone what happened—me, a teacher, school counselor, the police.

- If you are currently being sexually abused, don't protect the abuser any longer. Report the abuse. Talk to me, a teacher, your school counselor, or the police immediately.

- Don't drive around alone with people you've just met, especially older teens. Even harmless looking people can be trouble. Our world is a violent place today. Anyone, including you, could become someone's victim.

- Never take a ride home from school or work with a person you don't know, someone you've just met, a person with a bad reputation, or any person acting suspiciously.

- Follow your intuition. If something feels wrong, it probably is. Get out of the situation immediately.

- If you ever find yourself under attack, a hard blow with your knee or fist to the attacker's penis and scrotum can render him helpless for a few seconds so you can escape. A hard hit by both palms of the hands to the attacker's ears is another option. Taking a self-defense course through the local community center, YMCA, or YWCA should be a goal for all teens.

- When you leave school, a school activity, dance, or party with new friends or a new date, let another friend know what time you're leaving, where you're going, and with whom.

- Do not leave school, a school activity, dance, or party with someone you don't know or someone you've just met.

- Don't get in a situation where you are alone with people who have been drinking or doing drugs.

You and your friends can probably think of additional ways to guard against sexual abuse.

Incest, molestation, and rape are frightening experiences. They leave victims with confused feelings about themselves, sex, love, and relationships. There are people who can help. If you have been or know of someone who is being sexually abused, call your local county health clinic, local sexual abuse hot-line, or the national child abuse hot-line (800-422-4453). Professional mental health counselors are trained to help you rid yourself of the bad feelings and feel good again. It's important after any type of sexual abuse to talk with a counselor to help you resolve the trauma of the incident.

If you should ever be raped or abused, come to me or the police immediately. *Do not* shower, change clothes, or wipe down any part of your body. Obtaining a conviction on a rape is difficult unless the prosecutor has adequate hair, clothes fiber, and semen samples. Any of the perpetrator's hair, clothes fibers, and semen found on your body are evidence. I or the police will see that you're taken to a clinic or hospital where trained health care technicians will take the samples from you and then let you shower.

Michael, before I end this letter, there is one other important aspect of sexual abuse we must discuss; that aspect is *you*. As a male, you may have consensual sex with someone and still be accused of rape, abuse, or molestation.

## Protecting Yourself from Participating In or Being Accused of Abuse or Rape

You may find yourself in a situation where there is a potential for the people you are with to participate in some form of abuse or for you to be accused of abuse or rape. The following will help you avoid circumstances that might leave you open to someone's accusations.

* When dating or at parties, don't drink or do drugs. Drinking and drugs alter rational thought and heighten

aggressiveness. Being drunk or high can cause you to lose control.

* When making out is leading to intercourse, *any time* the girl says *stop*, or *no*, you must stop. Even if it's the very last second before the penis enters the vagina, or even if the penis is in the vagina. If the girl says *no* or *stop*, and you proceed against her will, you are committing rape. If this law seems harsh, consider if it were someone raping you? Wouldn't you want these same laws?

* Don't make out with girls who've been drinking or doing drugs. If a girl makes out with you or has sex with you, but then cries rape or abuse it will be her word against yours. Most people aren't dishonest, but these cases do happen.

* Some people don't realize how seductive their dress, body language, gestures, sexual comments, and flirting can be. A girl may think she is innocently flirting with a guy, but he interprets it as an invitation to have sex. When you date, ask questions and get answers. Never assume anything.

* Remember that in some states, sex with a female under age fourteen is considered rape, even if she consents.

* *Never* participate in, or encourage any type of group rape or abuse. Leave the situation and call 911 for help.

* Follow your intuition. If something feels wrong, it probably is. Get out of the situation immediately.

To avoid being accused of sexual abuse stay away from questionable sexual situations. Make the above your personal creed of sexual conduct.

Michael, while you were growing up, I tried to be alert to any sexual abuse. As a child I told you that no one (family member or anyone else) should ever touch the private parts of your body or play sex games with you. To my knowledge no one has. If I missed an incident, tell me or someone who can help. Get help now.

Michael, this letter is not intended to frighten you but to make you aware that sexual abuse is, unfortunately, a part of our society. Most of the relationships in your life will be healthy and good, but should you ever encounter sexual abuse, reread this letter and get help.

All my love,

Mom

_____

_____

_____

_____

_____

_____

_____

_____

_____

# LETTER 22

# MARRIAGE

Dear Michael,

I can't talk to you about sex and love without a letter on marriage. You may be saying, "Mom, marriage? Guys my age aren't even thinking about that stuff!"

Don't misunderstand me, Michael. I'm not pushing you to get married. If a couple is serious in high school, I think both partners should graduate and live on their own before marrying. Your life goals usually change significantly between age eighteen and twenty-five. But sometimes you date a girl during high school (perhaps you fall in love) and you begin thinking, "What if we were married someday?"

## High School Marriages
In high school your dating can become serious, in part, because your sexual feelings are intense. A few seventeen and eighteen year olds do fall in love, get married, and have good marriages. Be careful. What you take for love could be sexual lust. Sex alone won't keep a marriage together. One out of every two high school marriages end in divorce before five years of marriage.

High school marriages fall apart because people change after high school. Your goals change. Your outlook on life changes. Life is a lot different after graduation. You may swear you and your girlfriend won't change, but change happens.

In a marriage, when one partner grows and matures and the other doesn't and if other adjustments aren't made in the marriage, a split develops in the relationship that can lead to divorce.

But when you think you're in love, it's easy to become so absorbed in your girlfriend that you don't think rationally. The statistics show that the majority of men and women do not find their marriage partner in high school. Remember, only one percent of high school seniors find their life partner in high school.

Michael, if you and a girl become serious about marriage, please consider getting separate apartments after graduation. Date for a year before setting a wedding date. If your feelings for each other are real, they will grow stronger during that year.

I saw many of my friends marry right after high school. Within five years they divorced. The same thing happens today. People marry too early and for the wrong reasons.

## Are Both of You In Love and Is She the Right Girl?

Unfortunately, the love that leads to marriage is hard to describe. When it happens, you'll feel that this particular dating relationship is different. If you're both in love and thinking of marriage, you should both have a contented, peaceful feeling. But this feeling rarely happens on the first few dates; it builds as your relationship grows.

## How Do You Know When You're Both Ready for Marriage?

That's the tricky part. Throughout your life, you may fall in love more than once. But the girl you fall in love with may not be in love with you, or she may be in love but not ready to marry.

Your dad said there were two girls he thought of marrying. One wasn't in love with him; the other he married—me. It wouldn't have worked to marry the first girl because she didn't love him.

You'll both know you're ready to marry if, despite normal engagement jitters, you feel comfortable with the decision. It's better to cancel the wedding the day before than to go into a marriage with only one of you committed to it.

If you fall in love in high school, don't rush into marriage. Graduate, move out of the house, and date for a while. Have a long engagement to be sure that you are right for each other.

Approximately one in a hundred people find a husband or wife in high school. The majority of people don't marry until their twenties or thirties.

Before you marry, make sure that "you" or "your girlfriend" aren't marrying. . .

* to get out of the house or to quit school,

* for a father or mother figure to take care of you,

* for someone to love you,

* because it's the thing to do,

* thinking you'll learn to love your spouse later, or

* because it's great sex. Sex is only a small part of marriage and it won't keep a marriage together. But sex can easily trick you into thinking this person is the one!

Too many people marry for the wrong reasons or marry before they are ready. These marriages usually end in divorce. Do you know people who rushed into marriage and it didn't work?

On the following marriage checklist, mark the statements that apply to your relationship. Statements not checked should be talked about with your girlfriend and a compromise reached before you walk down the aisle.

☐ You both compromise to meet each other's needs and wants.

☐ You're at ease talking to each other. You're not putting on a false front for one another.

☐ You know each other's work, career, and personal goals. You're committed to supporting each other's goals.

☐ You both realize that marriage is a partnership and requires support from both partners for the rest of your lives.

☐ You know each other's views on religion, sex, money, marriage roles, male and female careers, economic status, family and child-rearing. You've talked through the compromises that are needed.

☐ You both enjoy some of the same interests, but you don't have to do everything together.

☐ You both know that a marriage needs affection to last. You're both comfortable expressing your affection—hugs, kisses, cuddles, and "I love yous." You aren't afraid to ask each other for a touch or big hug after a tough day.

☐ You both want to be married.

## The Realities of Marriage

Marriage is work. A marriage takes both partners to make it work. But when you love someone the work isn't as difficult and the rewards are great. However, marriage isn't without arguments, disagreements, trials, and pressures. Like the traditional vows tell us, marriage is for better or for worse, through good times and bad, through sickness and health.

During my marriage to your father, we've had a lot of money and no money; we've both been sick at times; we've both gone through job changes and age changes that were good and bad. But facing the good and bad together is what makes a twenty year marriage as strong, loving, and exciting as a first year marriage.

Don't marry thinking that once you are married you will change your partner's personality or habits. The number one mistake people make is thinking they can change their partner after marriage.

People can't change other people. A girl who is immature, selfish, demanding, rude, or lazy before marriage will be that way after marriage unless she changes herself. Do you want to put up with bad habits for the rest of your life? It is possible to love someone who would not make a good marriage partner.

*Mom,*

*How are my friends with divorced parents supposed to have good role models for marriage?*

Another good question, Michael. Many teens today have divorced parents. They can learn about marriage from their divorced parents by sitting down and talking to them. "Why did you and Dad (or you and Mom) marry? Why did you divorce? If you could redo the experience, what would you do differently?"

They can also read books on what makes marriage work, why people divorce, and how to know when a couple is ready for marriage. Just because teens have divorced parents doesn't mean that those teens can't have good marriages as adults.

## Divorce

Most people don't plan to divorce. But it happens and divorce hurts. It breaks up families and is hard on children. If people didn't rush into marriage so quickly, took the commitment of marriage seriously, and worked at their marriages once they were married, the divorce rate wouldn't be so high.

## Before You Marry

Be sure you and your girlfriend are both in love and committed to being married. Fall in love with your heart *and* your head.

During your engagement talk, talk, talk to each other. Usually couples are so taken by love, they don't discuss each other's views on the real issues of marriage—job goals, household chores, money, children, personal goals—until after the wedding ceremony. They say "I do," then find out later that their views about marriage are worlds apart.

Share with each other your expectations of what marriage will be like. Tell each other your future career, money, family, housing, and leisure goals. Do you know she likes to travel? Does she know you want to buy a speed boat? Is she a spender while you're a saver? Would you like her to always work outside the home, but she wants to stay home and be a full-time mom until the children are in school?

Understand fully each other's dreams, likes, and dislikes before you walk down the aisle. While your goals may change over the years, your marriage will have a better chance of success because you started with shared expectations.

## After You Marry

Once married, these housekeeping activities can help keep your marriage strong, happy, and healthy.

- Talk with each other daily. Don't let disagreements and disappointments fester. Practice forgiveness. No marriage is perfect, because people aren't perfect.

- Learn to laugh at yourself. Maintain a sense of humor about life and marriage.

- Commit to keeping your marriage alive and growing. Review that commitment to yourself morning and night.

- Nurture your love. Kiss each other good morning and good night. Hug and cuddle. There is nothing better than a spouse's warm, loving, hold-me-tight hug after a bad day.

- Regularly make time in your busy schedule to date each other and spend quality time together.

- Before going to sleep each night, hold each other and thank each other for the chores each of you do that become boring but keep the marriage moving—making dinner, washing clothes, repairing the car, diapering the children.

- Create a budget for yourselves. Include (1) a savings account, (2) a separate emergency savings, and (3) a weekly personal allowance for each of you. Work out the kinks in your new budget, then adjust that budget according to job and career changes.

- If serious problems arise over money, sex, careers, religion, children, or in-laws see a professional marriage counselor or mediator to help solve the problem and put your marriage back on track. There is no shame in seeing a counselor. Couples should work with marriage counselors at the first sign of trouble instead of waiting until the trouble has progressed to the point of divorce.

Marriage is compromise, an agreement to live your lives together, caring for and loving each other.

Marriage isn't a fairy-tale romance, a parent figure to take care of you, or you as the parent figure taking care of someone.

Good marriage partners are best friends, spouses, and lovers. You want to grow old together. You're a team, a pair, a couple.

I hope as an adult that you find someone you want to share your life with, and I wish you only the best.

All my love,

Mom

_____

_____

_____

_____

_____

_____

_____

_____

_____

_____

# Letter 23

# I Love You, Goodnight

Dear Michael,

This is my last letter in this collection. I hope I've given you information you can use to become comfortable with your sexuality, keep healthy, and make responsible dating decisions. If there are a few thoughts I would have you carry with you always, they are:

* Don't be afraid to be your own person. Love yourself for being you. Stand firm in your beliefs and values; remember that other people are entitled to their beliefs. Stand strong against peer pressure. Be your own man.

* Above everything else, finish high school. Then after high school obtain some type of on-the-job training, technical schooling, or college so you have a job skill to support yourself.

* Protect your sexuality. Your sexuality isn't something you pass around to everyone as if it were junk food to be eaten and you, the wrapper, thrown away.

* Take care of your body. If you do have sex before you marry, use condoms every time to protect yourself against STDs and pregnancy.

- Enjoy your teen years. If you date, great. If you don't date, that's fine too. Some people don't become interested in dating until after high school; they have a group of friends with whom they do things together.

Whenever you need to talk about anything—girls, sex, love, friendships, life—I am here for you. I will try to be a good listener, open-minded, and not judgmental. I'm also here if you just want a mom hug after a rotten day.

Michael, you're a wonderful young man. I wish you nothing but happiness. Even though we argue sometimes, as all moms and sons do, I will always love you and I'm proud to be your mom.

All my love,

Mom

_____

_____

_____

_____

_____

_____

_____

_____

_____

_____

_____

# Glossary of Terms

ABORTION. Termination of a pregnancy. There are two type of abortions; spontaneous abortion (miscarriage) and induced abortion. Spontaneous abortion occurs when the body naturally aborts the pregnancy because it cannot sustain the pregnancy. It usually happens before the twenty-fifth week of pregnancy. Induced abortion is a surgical procedure done by a licensed doctor when a woman chooses to terminate a pregnancy or when a pregnancy is endangering a woman's life and must be terminated.

ABSTINENCE. Not having intercourse. The only 100 percent effective method of not becoming pregnant or contracting many STDs.

ADOLESCENCE. The time period—normally between eleven and nineteen years of age—of a person's mental and physical maturing toward adulthood.

AFTERBIRTH. See placenta.

AIDS (Acquired Immune Deficiency Syndrome). STD. A deadly disease caused by a virus that attacks the body's immune system. AIDS is spread by contaminated body fluids and blood, usually through some type of intercourse or sharing unclean needles used to inject illegal drugs. Currently there is no known cure for AIDS. See also chart p. 150.

AMNIOCENTESIS. A test usually given to high-risk pregnant women (those over thirty years old or who were taking drugs or had an illness upon conception) to determine if the baby may have birth defects. The test is done by inserting a needle through the woman's belly into the baby's placenta and extracting a sample of amniotic fluid which is then examined for abnormalities.

ANAL INTERCOURSE. The insertion of the penis into the anus.

ARTIFICIAL INSEMINATION. Method of impregnation of a woman by insertion of sperm inside her vagina through a small tube. Artificial insemination is an option when regular intercourse does not result in pregnancy.

BIRTH CONTROL. Avoiding pregnancy by using contraceptive protection during each act of intercourse.

BIRTH DEFECTS. Medical problems that babies are born with such as under-developed limbs or internal organs, blindness and other problems. Birth defects may come from a variety of causes: defects in the ovum or sperm, inherited problems from either parent, the mother's exposure to harmful drugs or radiation during her pregnancy, the mother's body being too young to properly nourish the baby (teens having babies), premature births, and lack of oxygen to the baby during birth.

BISEXUAL. (slang: AC/DC) A person who engages in both heterosexual and homosexual relations.

BREASTS. Human mammary glands. The female breasts produce milk for the baby after childbirth. The male breast does not develop to accommodate milk production. Breasts are a source of sexual pleasure for most women and some men.

CAESAREAN SECTION. Surgical operation (making an incision through a mother's abdomen and the wall of her uterus) to deliver a baby when vaginal delivery is not an option.

CERVIX. Opening to the uterus located at the top of the vagina.

CHANCROID. STD. (See chart p. 150)

CHILDBIRTH. The process in which a baby is pushed out of the woman's uterus and vaginal canal when it is ready to be born.

CHILD MOLESTER. Person who inappropriately fondles children and teens, and/or has sexual relations with them.

CHLAMYDIA. STD. (See chart p. 150)

CHROMOSOMES. Portions of the ovum and sperm that contain genetic information for such characteristics as hair color, bone structure, skin color, eye color, and sex.

CIRCUMCISION. A surgical procedure dating back to biblical days to remove the loose flap or foreskin covering the end of the male penis. Circumcision is usually performed within twenty-four hours of a healthy birth.

CLIMAX. See Orgasm.

CLITORIS (Slang; clit). A small, nerve sensitive pleasure organ located in the soft folds of skin just above the females urinary and vaginal openings. Stimulating the clitoris through masturbation, oral sex, or intercourse is the way most women achieve orgasm.

COITUS. Another name for sexual intercourse.

CONCEPTION. The uniting of ovum and sperm. Fertilization of a female egg by the male sperm.

CONDOMS (rubbers, prophylactics). Contraceptive device of thin latex rubber that fits on the penis and holds the semen during intercourse.

CONTRACEPTION. The prevention of pregnancy. Various methods used such as condoms , the pill, and diaphragm.

CUNNILINGUS. The male orally stimulates the female's external sex organs.

DIAPHRAGM. Form of birth control. The diaphragm is a soft rubber disk with a flexible rim that is used with contraceptive cream or jelly. It is inserted into the vagina so that it covers the cervix. It is a prescription contraceptive and must be fitted by a doctor.

DOUCHE. A homemade or commercially prepared solution of filtered water and other ingredients that rinses and cleanses the vagina. Not recommended unless used under doctor's orders because douching can harm the vagina's natural acidity balance.

EJACULATION. When an erect penis releases semen and sperm through intercourse, masturbation, or wet dreams.

EMBRYO. A human organism from forty-eight hours after conception to the end of the eighth week of development.

ERECTION (slang: hard-on, boner). Temporary hardening or stiffening of the penis caused by increased blood flow to the spongy tissue inside the penis. Generally, erections are caused by sexual thoughts or stimulation, but spontaneous erections happen for no particular reason.

ESTROGEN. Hormone produced by the female ovary gland. Maintains female secondary sex characteristics.

EXHIBITIONIST. A person who exposes her or his sexual organs in public.

FALLOPIAN TUBES. Small slender tubes about the size of spaghetti that connect a female's ovaries to her uterus.

FELLATIO. The female orally stimulates the male's penis.

FETUS. Unborn human from eight weeks of development to birth.

FOREPLAY. Affectionate kissing, hugging, and caressing/stimulating sexual organs between partners prior to sexual intercourse.

FORESKIN. Hood-like piece of skin covering the tip of the uncircumcised penis.

FRATERNAL TWINS. Two separate ovum are fertilized and grow in the uterus. Fraternal twins may not have identical looks and they can be same sex twins or opposite sex twins.

FRENCH KISSING (tongue kissing). While kissing, a person puts her or his tongue in the other person's mouth. French kissing includes using the tip of the tongue or the entire tongue.

GAY. Another term for male homosexuals; sometimes used to describe both male and female homosexuals.

GENETIC. Pertaining to hereditary characteristics transferred from parents to children by way of chromosomes found in sperm and ova.

GENITALIA. (genitals). Human external sex organs.

GENITAL WARTS. STD. (See chart p. 150)

GESTATION. Period of carrying off spring in the uterus from conception to birth.

GLANS. Head of penis.

GONORRHEA. STD. (See chart p. 151)

HEMORRHOIDS. Irritating and sometimes painful, swollen vein clusters outside or inside your anus (rectum). Minor hemorrhoids can be treated with non-prescription hemorrhoids creams, warm baths, exercise, proper diet to maintain proper weight and normal bowel movements. Child birth and strenuous exercise are frequent causes.

HEPATITIS (Type B). STD. (See chart p. 151)

HERPES. A common STD (viral) which can cause harm to mother and baby. Herpes usually appears in the form of sores on the genitals. (Also see p. 151).

HETEROSEXUAL. Person who is sexually attracted to persons of the opposite sex—males attracted to females, females to males.

HOMOSEXUAL. Person who is sexually attracted to members of her or his same sex.

HORMONE. A substance produced in one part of the body and transported by bodily fluids to another part of the body where it has a specific effect.

HYMEN. Thin piece of skin that may block or partially block the vaginal opening. Hymen structure varies greatly and some women are born without hymens.

HYSTERECTOMY. Surgery that removes a female's uterus and/or the ovaries and fallopian tubes for health reasons such as severe menstrual problems and pre-cancerous cell detection.

IDENTICAL TWIN. The fertilized ovum splits creating two separate same sex, identical-looking embryos. Twins are usually born within a few minutes of each other.

INCEST. Any sexual activity (including oral sex or intercourse) between family members other than husband-wife sexual relations. Incest is a crime. Incest most often occurs between parent and child or between siblings.

INFERTILITY (sterility). In women, the inability to become pregnant; in men the inability to produce sufficient sperm for conception.

IUD (Intrauterine device). See chart p. 157.

LABIA (lips). The two flaps of skin on each side of the vaginal opening.

LESBIAN. Another name for female homosexual. A female who is sexually attracted to other females.

MAKING OUT (necking). Prolonged kissing sessions.

MASOCHISM. A degrading sexual exploitation in which a person receives pleasure from being abused or dominated by another person (masochist—the person suffering).

MASTURBATION (slang: jacking, jerking or beating off, playing with yourself, beating your meat). Self-stimulating one's clitoris or penis, usually to the point of orgasm.

MENARCHE. Medical term for a girl's first menstruai period.

MENSES. Blood and dead cells discharged from the uterus through the vagina each month during menstruation.

MENSTRUATION (slang: period, on the rag). Monthly shedding of unfertilized ovum and uterine lining of non-pregnant females.

MISCARRIAGE. See Abortion.

NOCTURNAL EMISSION (wet dream). Semen released from the penis while a male is asleep.

ORAL SEX (cunnilingus, fellatio—slang: blow job, 69ing, giving head, eating at the y). A form of sexual expression in which one person stimulates another person's sexual organs by using her or his mouth and tongue.

ORGASM (climax—slang: cuming/coming). The moment of sexual stimulation when the nerve endings in the penis or clitoris register an eruption of pleasurable feeling.

OVARIES. Sex glands in the female where ova are stored.

OVARIAN CYST. An abnormal growth of cells on an ovary. Usually treated by high-estrogen contraceptives to shrink the growth or removed by surgery. Symptoms may include mild to severe abdominal pain and missed periods.

PENIS. Male sex organ that releases urine from the bladder and also deposits sperm in the female vagina during intercourse.

PHALLIC SYMBOL. Term used to refer to any object, shaped like an erect penis.

PLACENTA (afterbirth). Spongy mass of blood and tissue nurturing the embryo and fetus during development; expelled after birth of baby.

PMS (premenstrual syndrome). A group of physical and emotional symptoms that precede a menstrual period, such as fluid retention, fatigue, irritability, depression, and headache.

PORNOGRAPHY. Sexually explicit written or visual material created for the purpose of sexual stimulation or sexual perversion.

PREGNANCY. In human females the condition of a fertilized ovum attached to the uterus and period a developing fetus is carried within the uterus.

PROGESTERONE. A female hormone, also synthetically produced for contraceptive use in the Pill.

PROSTATE GLAND. Male sex gland that produces semen.

PUBERTY. Growth stage (usually between ages ten to nineteen) in which a person's child body develops into their adult body including the maturing of their reproductive system.

PUBIC HAIR. Male and female hair in the external genital area.

PUBIC LICE. STD. (See chart p. 151)

RAPE. A sex crime punishable by law in which a person forces another person to have intercourse.

S & M. Abbreviation for sadism and masochism.

SADISM. Degrading sexual exploitation in which a person receives pleasure from sexually abusing or domination another person (sadist—person inflicting the pain).

SADOMASOCHISM. Degrading sexual exploitation in which a person receives pleasure from inflicting sexual pain on oneself and others.

SCROTUM. Sac of skin that houses the male testicles.

SEMEN. Sticky white liquid containing sperm. It is ejaculated from the penis during intercourse, masturbation, or wet dreams.

SEXUAL INTERCOURSE (copulating, coupling—slang: making love, doing it, going all the way, screwing, fucking, humping, poking). Insertion of the erect male penis into the female's vagina.

SIAMESE TWINS. Twins whose bodies are physically joined together at birth—a rare occurrence.

SPERM. Male reproductive cell that fertilizes the female's ovum (female reproductive cell) for the creation of new human life.

SPERMICIDE. Sperm-killing chemical in contraceptive foams, cremes and jellies to kill sperm, thus preventing conception.

SPONTANEOUS ERECTION. Uncontrollable erection of the penis for no apparent reason.

STDs (sexually transmitted diseases). Harmful diseases that are transmitted from one partner to another by sexual contact (vaginal, oral, and anal).

STILLBIRTH. A baby that is born dead because of a malfunction in development or delivery. With good prenatal care, stillbirths rare.

SYPHILIS. STD. (See chart p. 151)

TESTOSTERONE. The male sex hormone.

TRANSVESTITE. A person who enjoys wearing the other sex's clothing.

TRICHOMONIASIS. STD. (See chart p. 151)

TOXIC SHOCK SYNDROME (TSS). A rare but serious, sometimes fatal disease caused by improper use of tampons.

TUBAL LIGATION. Surgery in which a female's fallopian tubes are tied so ova and sperm can't unite. This is a permanent form of contraception.

UTERUS (womb). Muscular, pear-shaped, sex organ in the female that houses the fetus as it grows and develops.

VAGINA (slang: cunt, pussy, box, hole, snatch). Passageway of tough elastic muscle leading from the external genitalia to the uterus.

VAGINITIS. An itching or burning inflammation of the vagina and vulva which can be caused by a variety of disorders including yeast infections and STDs.

VASECTOMY. Permanent contraceptive method for men who do not want to father any/or more children; surgery where the vas deferens is cut to prevent sperm from mixing with the semen.

VENEREAL DISEASE. See STD.

VIRGIN. Man or woman who has not experienced sexual intercourse.

VULVA. External genital organs of female.

WET DREAM. See Nocturnal Emission.

WITHDRAWAL. The male pulling his penis out of the female's vagina before ejaculation—withdrawal is not a form of birth control. Pulling out is useless since sperm from pre-ejaculatory semen from the end of the penis is already in the vagina.

WOMB. See Uterus.

# Additional Reading

Acker, Loren, Ph.D. *Aids Proofing Your Kids: A Step by Step Guide*. Hillsboro, Oregon: Beyond Words Publishing Company, 1992.

Bell, Ruth. *Changing Bodies, Changing Lives: A Book for Teens on Sex and Relationships*. New York: Random House, 1987.

Fairchild, Betty, and Nancy Hayward. *Now That You Know: What Every Parent Should Know About Homosexuality*. Updated ed. San Diego: Harcourt Brace Jovanovich, 1989.

Ford, Michael Thomas. *One Hundred Questions and Answers About AIDS: A Guide for Young People*. Parisspany, NJ: New Discovery Books, 1992.

Harris, Robie H. *It's Perfectly Normal: Changing Bodies, Growing Up, Sex and Sexual Health*. Cambridge, MA: Candlewick Press, 1994.

Heron, Ann (editor). *Two Teenagers in Twenty: Writings by Gay and Lesbian Youth*. Boston: Alyson Publications, 1994.

Madaras, Lynda. *The What's Happening To My Body? Book for Boys: A Growing Up Guide for Parents and Sons*. New York: Newmarket Press, rev. 1991.

Miller, Patricia Martins, *Sex is Not a Four-Letter Word! Talking Sex with Your Children Made Easier*. New York: The Crossroad Publishing Company, 1995.

Riera, Michael, Ph.D. *Uncommon Sense for Parents with Teenagers.* Berkeley, CA: Celestial Arts, 1995.

Rush, Florence. *The Best Kept Secret: Sexual Abuse of Children.* New York: McGraw-Hill Book Company, 1991.

Short, Ray E. *Sex, Love or Infatuation: How Can I Really Know?* Minneapolis, MN: Augsburg Fortress, 1990.

Tribe, Lawrence H. *Abortion; the Clash of Absolutes.* New York: Norton, rev. 1992.

Weisman, Michael and Betsy. *What We Told Our Kids About Sex.* New York: Harcourt Brace Jovanovich, 1987.

# Index

# About the Author

Cynthia G. Akagi is a Certified Family Life Educator (CFLE) and holds a master's degree in human development and family life education. She consults with school districts and communities, presents *Love vs. Sex* seminars at schools, and teaches sexuality education classes and workshops. Ms. Akagi is also the author of *Dear Larissa: Sexuality Education for Girls Ages 11-17*, a companion book to *Dear Michael*. She and her husband have two children, a son and a daughter.